CATTLE LAMENESS AND HOOFCARE
An Illustrated Guide

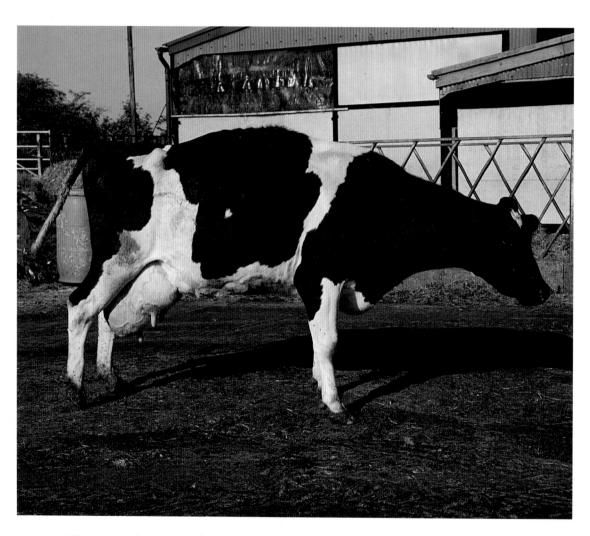

The typical stance of a cow with generalised lameness and laminitis.

CATTLE LAMENESS AND HOOFCARE
An Illustrated Guide

Roger Blowey
B.Sc., B.V.Sc., FRCVS

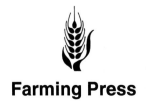

Farming Press

First published 1993
Reprinted with alterations 1998

Copyright © Roger Blowey 1993

German translation: Verlag Eugen Ulmer GmbH & Co.
Japanese translation: Tuttle-Mori Agency Ltd

A catalogue record for this book is available from the British Library

ISBN 0 85236 252 8

Published by Farming Press
Miller Freeman plc
Wharfedale Road, Ipswich IP1 4LG, United Kingdom

Distributed in North America
by Diamond Farm Enterprises,
Box 537, Alexandria Bay, NY 13607, USA

Illustrations by Jane Upton

Cover design by Andrew Thistlethwaite
Set by Galleon Typesetters, Ipswich
Printed and bound in Great Britain by Butler and Tanner Ltd, Frome and London

Contents

Foreword

A lot has happened in modern dairy husbandry during the last 25 years. Changes in housing, feeding etc. have been enormous and these have had their effect on dairy cows, not least on milk yield. Farmers these days ask a lot more from their cows.

Therefore management on the farm becomes more and more important. The farmer himself can minimise foot disease and foot problems by feeding his cows sensibly, maintaining clean and dry housing, using foot-baths, and by sound breeding. One major aspect of management, described in this book, is hoofcare.

I like to emphasise the need for preventive foot trimming. It is a well-known fact that claws overgrow and eventually cause lameness by sole ulcers, white line defects etc. If hoofcare is carried out regularly, ulceration of the sole can be prevented. If the quick becomes bruised, the cow will change its posture and gait in order to relieve pain. This can be recognised by the farmer and is a good reason to trim the feet. Prevention is better than cure.

In the Netherlands it is accepted that cows' feet should be regularly trimmed, e.g. twice each year, preferably in spring and in autumn. Even so, laminitis remains a difficult condition requiring a lot of attention. Individual cases are hard to prevent where there is a herd problem. In his book Roger Blowey gives a good picture of foot diseases and how to deal with and prevent them.

I have read the book with pleasure and feel that it can significantly contribute to proper footcare on farms.

Pieter Kloosterman, Teacher in Hoofcare Dairy Training Centre Friesland (DTC-Friesland), Oenkerk, The Netherlands

Acknowledgements

All the photographs in this book have been taken on farms in the course of my day-to-day general practice and I would like, once again, to acknowledge the patience and understanding of the many Gloucestershire farmers who waited, often at the most inconvenient times, while I went away to get my camera! This book is dedicated to them.

Special thanks must go to Jane Upton, for her excellent preparation of the diagrams, and to Catherine Girdler, who so proficiently tackled the typing of the manuscript. Both have made a major contribution towards this book.

I would also like to acknowledge the help of Bob Ward for instructive discussions, David Logue, Susan Kempson, Janet O'Connell and David Pepper for the use of their material, the staff at Farming Press for their patience and help during the preparation of this book, and of course Pieter Kloosterman who has so kindly read the manuscript and written the Foreword. Thanks are due to the Veterinary Record and Wolfe Publications who have published some of the photographs previously in *In Practice, A Colour Atlas of Diseases and Disorders of Cattle* and *Self-Assessment Tests in Veterinary Medicine*. Finally, thanks must go to my wife, Norma, for continued tolerance, patience and support.

Dedicated to My Parents

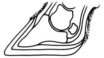

CHAPTER ONE

The Incidence and Costs
of Lameness

Lameness, as every farmer knows, is a major cost to the dairy herd. This 'cost' has three main components: the economic losses resulting from reduced production; the labour costs associated with the treatment and husbandry of chronically lame animals; and the welfare costs of suffering to the individual affected cow. Lameness is undoubtedly a major welfare problem. It is also the condition which accounts for the third largest loss of income in the dairy herd, dwarfed only by mastitis and poor fertility. At worst, affected cows have to be culled. This increases overall culling rates and hence replacement costs. In those cows which can be treated, there is often a dramatic weight loss, milk yield falls and, in protracted cases in early lactation, fertility is affected. In addition, there will be the costs of treatment, whether on-farm labour is used or veterinary attention is sought. If antibiotics are administered milk may have to be discarded.

One of the most dramatic changes seen in lame cows is undoubtedly weight loss. It is surprising how many cows continue to milk, especially in the early stages of lameness, but weight loss can be dramatic. Farmers who have out-of-parlour computer feeders have often commented that reduced concentrate intake is seen some 24 hours before lameness is noticed.

In a recent study (*30, 60*)* of grazing animals, it was shown that lame cows spent longer lying down and less time grazing and even when they did graze, bite rates were lower. Lame cows lose the ability to defend themselves and get pushed further down the scale of 'social dominance'. They tend to be later entering the milking parlour and more restless in

* Bracketed numbers refer to references which are found on pages 77-79.

1

the parlour than non-lame animals.

Not surprisingly, fertility is also affected. A detailed study of 427 cases of lameness in 17 dairy herds in Somerset (*19*) showed that affected cows took between 0 and 40 days (an average of 14 days) longer to get back in calf, depending on the stage of lactation when the cow was first affected, the cause of the lameness and its severity. Some cows did not recover, of course, and hence culling rates were increased. Yields were depressed by between 1 and 20%, depending on the severity of the lameness.

A late lactation cow with a mild case of foul in the foot or digital dermatitis is easily treated and suffers virtually no adverse effects. A severe, penetrating ulcer with secondary infection of the navicular bursa or pedal joint can lead to the loss of the cow and obviously a substantial loss of income.

The incidence of lameness varies between farms, with quoted figures for well-recorded herds varying between 4 and 55% (*56*). This wide variation partly arises from the source of the survey material. If veterinary practice records are used, then a lower incidence is obtained (4.7 – 5.5%) (*24, 55*). However, taking combined veterinary and farm treatments gives an annual incidence of approximately 25% of cows in the national herd being treated for lameness each year (*3, 61*). This incidence has persisted over several years in the late eighties and early nineties (*35*). Considerably more cows than this need corrective hoof-trimming.

A survey carried out in the late seventies (*55*) showed that leg disorders accounted for only 12% of the total number of cases of lameness recorded and these were mainly calving injuries. This means that 88% of lameness was associated with the foot. Of these, the majority (86%) were in the hind feet, with the outer claw (85%) being the most likely to be affected. As front feet are much more difficult to restrain and treat, perhaps it is just as well that they are not so commonly involved!

In an assessment of the losses associated with lameness, Esslemont (*25*) estimated that lameness cost the dairy industry in England and Wales £90 million per year (1990 values) or £31.50 for every cow in your herd! He also estimated that the average cost of lameness in a typically affected cow was £227 – £297 for a sole ulcer, £139 – £153 for digital disease (white line infection, sole abscess or sole penetration), and £24 – £58 for interdigital disease (foul, dermatitis, skin hyperplasia, etc.), the major proportion of these costs arising from the effects of lameness in early lactation on subsequent fertility and culling rates. These figures do not take into account the welfare of the cow, nor the additional work and frustration caused to the herdsman in the treatment, husbandry and management of such cows.

So, what can be done about this expensive disease? The objectives of this book are to give the reader a better understanding of the anatomy of the foot and the importance of its weight-bearing surfaces; to see what happens during overgrowth and how this results in the foot becoming destabilised; to discuss and demonstrate the principles of foot-trimming; to describe and illustrate the various causes of lameness; and, finally, to examine some of the more important aspects of lameness prevention.

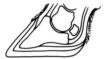

CHAPTER TWO

Foot Structure and Function and Laminitis

THE STRUCTURE OF THE FOOT

Many technical terms will be used throughout this book. This is in an attempt to increase the precision of the descriptions and is certainly not intended to confuse the reader. By initially explaining and defining the terms and then by using them repeatedly throughout the text, it is hoped that they will become easily understood and part of 'comfortable' language.

The foot consists of two separate digits, the outer or lateral claw and the inner or medial claw. Figure 2.1 shows a bovine right hind foot, viewed from the bottom and from the side. Note how the lateral claw is slightly larger than the medial. In front feet this is reversed, with the medial claw being larger than the lateral. The outer wall of each claw is known as the abaxial surface and the inner wall, facing the space between the claws, is the axial surface. The space between the claws is known as the interdigital cleft and this separates the two heel bulbs. The front surface of the foot, at the toe, is known as the anterior aspect and the rear, at the heel, the posterior aspect.

The two claws are highly modified forms of the second and third human fingers (Figure 2.2), where the nail forms a complete covering around the finger tip. The first and fourth fingers are equivalent to the accessory digits, and the thumb has totally disappeared.

The claw consists of three basic tissue components (Figure 2.3). Starting from the outside these are:

- hoof, the hard outer casing of the foot
- corium or quick, a support structure containing nerves and blood vessels and carrying nutrients for hoof formation
- pedal bone, navicular bone and their associated structures

3

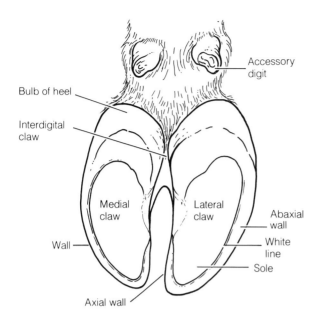

FIGURE 2.1 Diagram of right hind foot viewed from the bottom (above) and from the side (below), giving the nomenclature of its surfaces.

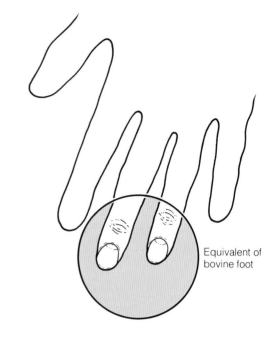

FIGURE 2.2 The human hand compared to the bovine foot.

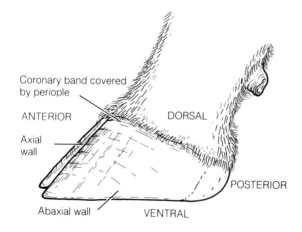

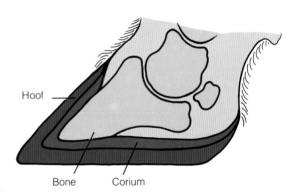

FIGURE 2.3 The three basic tissues of the foot: hoof, corium and bone.

The horn of the hoof is the extensively modified superficial layer of the skin (technically known as the epidermis) which has become expanded and impregnated with a hardener known as keratin. The corium is equivalent to the dermis or lower part of the skin and provides nutrition for the hoof, although it does not secrete or produce the hoof.

Technical texts subdivide the hoof and the corium into various layers. These are listed below for reference.

Hoof (epidermis):

- stratum corneum
- stratum granulosum
- stratum spinosum
- stratum germinativum

4

Basement membrane (the junction between the epidermis and the corium)

Corium (dermis):

- stratum lamellatum (laminae) or papillarae (papillae)
- stratum vasculosum
- stratum periostale (periosteum)

THE HOOF

The hoof can be subdivided into four component areas:

- the periople
- the wall
- the sole
- the heel

The Periople

The periople is the hairless band of soft horn which separates the hoof wall from the skin at the coronary band and is clearly seen in Plate 2.1. It is continuous from one claw to the other and merges with the bulb of the heel. The periople is responsible for the smooth, waxy coating seen over the front of good quality hooves. Its function is to prevent excess water loss and hence keep the foot supple. Unfortunately, it deteriorates with age and with hot dry sandy conditions underfoot. When perioplic horn is damaged, for example, during very dry weather, the hoof wall may crack, producing a vertical fissure, more commonly known as a sandcrack (see Plate 5.46).

The Wall

The wall of the hoof is formed at the papillae, small finger-like projections of the corium, sited just below the coronary band. Figure 2.4 and Plates 2.2 and 2.4 show how the wall is thinner at this point. The papillae are covered by the stratum germinativum, or germinative layer, of the epidermis. This is the basic microscopic layer which is responsible for horn formation.

These cells are then filled with a sulphur-containing hardener (the onychogenic substance) which matures in the stratum spinosum to produce keratin, an extremely hard substance. Maturation of keratin involves the oxidation of the sulphur-containing amino acid cysteine to form cystine. The majority of the hoof wall consists of the stratum corneum, the mature, hardened layer. Keratin is also

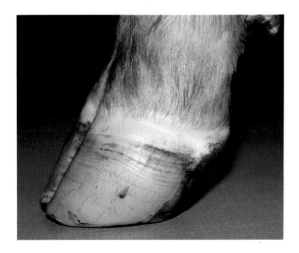

PLATE 2.1 *Lateral view of the claw, showing the periople and steep angle of the anterior hoof wall.*

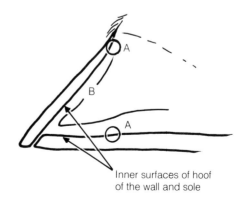

Inner surfaces of hoof
of the wall and sole

FIGURE 2.4   A section of the hoof showing: A. papillae at the site of horn formation; B. laminae.

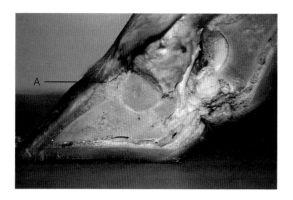

PLATE 2.2 *Transverse section of the foot. Note how the hoof wall is thinner in the region of the papillae, just below the coronary band (A). The thick, glistening white flexor tendon runs down the rear of the navicular bone to attach to the base of the pedal bone.*

present in hair, in the enamel of teeth and, to a lesser extent, in the superficial layers of our skin.

To increase its strength, the cells of the hoof are arranged in a series of pipes or tubules, the growth of each tubule being effectively an extrusion process from the papilla (Figure 2.5).

Horn tubules are glued together by further keratin-containing cells originating from the sides and base of the papillae to produce intertubular horn (Figure 2.5).

The tubules run longitudinally down the front of the hoof and vertically down through the sole. Intertubular horn is softer than tubular horn, but the number of horn tubules in a hoof is fixed at birth. This means that as a hoof gets larger, it does so by an expansion of intertubular horn and hence a very large, flat foot in a cow is generally softer and weaker than the small, compact hoof of a heifer.

Once formed, the wall passes slowly down over the front of the foot, at a rate of approximately 5mm per month. As the distance from the coronary band to the wearing surface at the toe is approximately 75mm, this means that the horn will not come into wear until 15 months after it has been produced (75mm divided by 5mm per month).

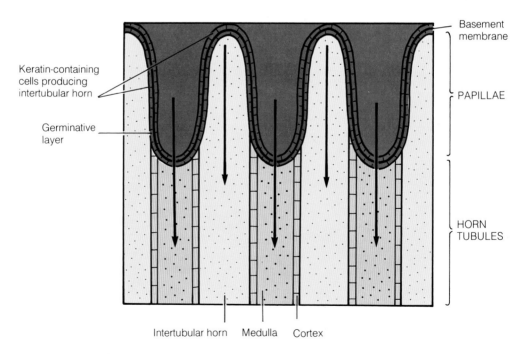

FIGURE 2.5 Detailed structure of the papillae, producing horn tubules and intertubular horn.

6

The hoof wall needs to be firmly attached to the underlying structures which it protects and yet, at the same time, it must have a small amount of movement in order to act as a shock absorber during locomotion. These dual functions are achieved by a series of interdigitating leaves, known as the laminae, which run down the inside of the hoof wall. Plate 2.3 is a boiled-out specimen of a hoof which shows the laminae very well. There are some 1,300 laminae in total, arranged like the gills of a fish, and all are present at birth.

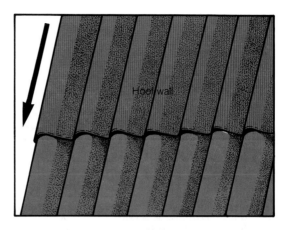

FIGURE 2.6 A diagrammatic representation of laminae — one sheet of corrugated cardboard sliding over another.

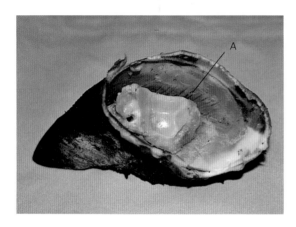

PLATE 2.3   A boiled out specimen of the hoof, showing pink laminae running down the inside of the hoof wall (A) and the position of the pedal bone inside the hoof.

The movement of the hoof wall down over the laminae has been compared to one piece of corrugated cardboard (the wall) moving down a second, stationary piece (Figure 2.6). The corrugations of the laminae are much deeper than those of the cardboard, of course, giving much greater support and adhesion.

The Sole

The horn of the sole is formed from papillae on the sole and hence consists of horn tubules and an intertubular matrix (Figure 2.7). There are no laminae in the sole and the solar horn grows directly downwards from beneath the pedal bone. Where the horn of the wall meets the horn of the sole there is a cemented junction, known as the white line. This can be clearly seen in Plates 2.4, 2.6 and 4.8. It runs from the bulb of the heel to the toe and then back along the first third of the axial wall, until the wall no longer becomes a weight-bearing surface. Being a junction, it is a point of weakness and a common site for impaction of debris and entry of infection.

Why is the white line white? This is probably because movement of the wall over the laminae is achieved by the laminae producing small quantities of horn, sometimes known as the laminar horn leaflet cells (40). Their position is shown diagrammatically in Figure 2.7. The horn leaflets produced by the laminae consist of long, thin cells, running parallel with one another (Figure 2.8). Where the laminae of the wall end and the papillae of the sole start, there is a small intermediate area which produces 'interdigitating horn', that is horn which connects the wall to the sole. This consists of flat, irregular-shaped cells, again containing keratin

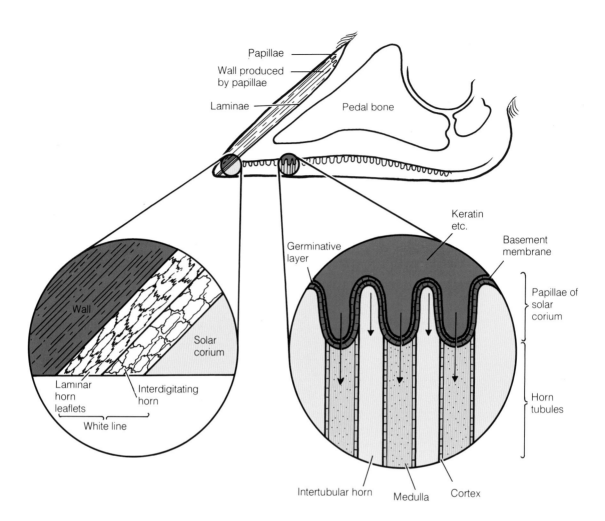

FIGURE 2.7   The structure of the hoof wall, sole and white line.

(Figure 2.9). There are no horn tubules in this part of the white line and this, combined with the shape of the interdigitating horn cells, is thought to account for both the inherent weakness of the area and also for its ability to move slightly during weightbearing, returning to its original shape when at rest (36).

We have already seen how the process of keratinisation (hardening) starts in the inner layer of the hoof, but full maturation of keratin does not occur until it reaches the outer layers (the stratum corneum). The lower levels of the laminae are also non-pigmented. The white line

therefore consists of immature laminar horn leaflets joined to the sole by interdigitating horn. This immature horn is non-pigmented and hence the term **white** line. It is also keratinised incompletely, and therefore considerably weaker. The distinct junction of the wall with the horn of the white line is clearly seen in Plate 2.4.

The Heel

The heel, or bulb of the hoof, is a rounded area covered by softer horn, a continuation of the perioplic layer. Being

8

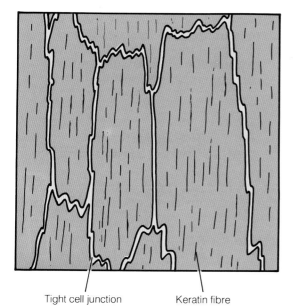

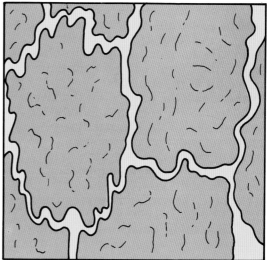

Tight cell junction   Keratin fibre

FIGURE 2.8   Well organised, elongated squame cells from laminar leaflet horn. Keratin fibres are straight and the cell junctions are tight. *(D. Logue and S. Kempson)*

FIGURE 2.9   Rounded squame cells from interdigitating horn. Keratin is present, but the fibres are not elongated. *(D. Logue and S. Kempson)*

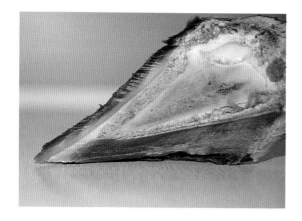

PLATE 2.4   Transverse section of the hoof. The white of the white line and its junction with the hoof wall are clearly visible.

flexible, the heel compresses during weightbearing and returns to normal when pressure is removed. These continual changes in shape put considerable pressure on the adjacent, more rigid hoof wall however. This has

been suggested as a reason why white line disease (impaction and infection) is more common in the abaxial (outer) wall at the sole – heel junction (site 1, Figure 5.1) than elsewhere in the foot (*48*).

THE CORIUM

The second tissue within the claw is the corium or quick and is the modified dermis of the skin (the hoof is the modified epidermis). The corium is the support tissue of the foot. It contains nerves and blood vessels for the hoof and the pedal bone and it carries the nutrients required for horn formation and for feeding the periosteum which surrounds the pedal bone. While the horn of the hoof is dead, the corium is very much alive. When damaged it will bleed and cause pain.

The corium totally lines the inside of the hoof, as shown in Figure 2.3 and Plates 2.2 and 2.4. Towards the coronary band it is modified, to form the finger-like projections known as papillae which

9

penetrate like pegs into the overlying horn. The epidermis covering these papillae is the basic structure which produces the horn of the hoof. The blood vessels of the corium carry the nutrients required for horn formation.

Further down the wall, below the layer of the papillae, the corium is modified to form the leaves of the laminae. These interdigitate with the corresponding laminae of the hoof, to provide a tough but suspensory system for supporting the bodyweight of the cow.

At the heel, the corium is impregnated with fat, fibrous and elastic tissue, to form the digital cushion. Small areas of yellow elastic tissue can be seen in Plate 2.2. The digital cushion acts as an extremely important shock absorber during weightbearing and locomotion. Being covered by the flexible heel horn, it can be compressed, thus preventing jarring of the skeleton. When no longer weightbearing, it returns to its original shape.

Maintenance of adequate bloodflow within the foot is extremely important for horn formation and yet when the animal's weight is borne by its feet, blood flow is difficult. There are three main mechanisms involved:

- The digital cushion acts as a pump to suck blood out of the foot and force it back into circulation. In the hind foot especially, the heel makes contact with the ground first and this initiates the pumping action. Clearly lack of exercise impedes circulation.
- The minute blood vessels (the capillaries) in the corium expand and contract by muscle action as weight is borne by the feet. This muscle activity is destroyed by toxins in laminitis.
- There are by-pass mechanisms, known as arteriovenous shunts, which when weightbearing occurs, enable blood to circulate across the top of the foot, rather than through the capillaries of the corium. However, when the corium has been damaged by laminitis

(especially in horses) the shunt may remain open too long, leading to pooling of blood in the capillaries, poor oxygenation of the tissues and consequently poor horn formation.

THE BONES AND ASSOCIATED STRUCTURES

The third tissue, deep within the foot, is the pedal bone and associated structures.

Pedal Bone

The major bone is the pedal bone, equivalent to the very last bone in our fingertip (Figure 2.2), and is technically referred to as the third phalangeal bone. The pedal bone fits well forward in the hoof, being separated from the horn at the toe by quite a thin layer of corium. Laminae are more numerous over the anterior (front) and abaxial (outer) walls of the hoof and hence the pedal bone is essentially suspended within the hoof at these points. This 'tight fit' towards the toe is clearly shown in Figure 2.3 and the area of attachment to the laminae of the abaxial wall can be seen in Plate 2.3. When the cow walks there is therefore relatively little movement of the pedal bone at the toe and on the abaxial wall, but posteriorly towards the heel and also axially towards the interdigital cleft the amount of movement is greater.

In addition, in the lateral (outer) claw the pedal bone rests partly on the sole, while in the medial claw it is more tightly attached to the wall and thus exerts less pressure on the sole when weightbearing (58).

This could be one reason why there is a higher proportion of sole ulcers in the lateral claws of hind feet. In addition, there are stretching and depressing forces between the laminae and the hoof wall during walking (25). These forces are greatest on the abaxial wall of the lateral claw, particularly at a point halfway between the coronary band and the sole and posteriorly towards the heel. It has been proposed (25) that these forces are responsible for the increased incidence of white line separation and abscessation at this point (site 1, Figure 5.1).

The pedal bone only extends to about three-quarters of the distance to the heel and the rear edge of the pedal bone sits almost directly above the sole ulcer site, as can be seen in Plate 2.2 and in the boiled-out specimen in Plate 2.3.

Figure 2.10 shows how weight transmitted down the leg can cause pinching of the corium between the hard surfaces of the rear edge of the pedal bone and the horn of the sole beneath.

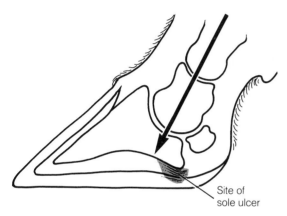

Site of sole ulcer

FIGURE 2.10   Weight passing down the leg will be partially transmitted onto the posterior (rear) edge of the pedal bone and this could cause pinching and damage to the corium.

The effect is exacerbated by the arched shape of the lower edge of the pedal bone, especially on its axial (inner) surface. This is also where its attachment to the hoof is minimal and movement will therefore be greater. The shape of the pedal bone is clearly seen in Plate 2.5. (Holes in the pedal bone allow the entry of blood vessels.) The pinching between pedal bone and hoof damages blood vessels in the corium, releasing blood cells which are then mixed with new hoof as it is formed.

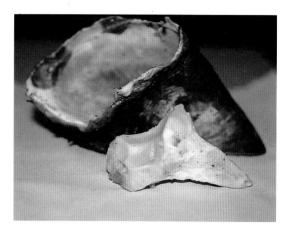

PLATE 2.5   A boiled out specimen showing the pedal bone with the arch on the axial aspect. Excess weight on the rear edge of the pedal bone could lead to bruising or a sole ulcer.

Eventually the mixture of blood and hoof grows to the surface of the sole. Plates 2.6 and 2.7 are typical examples.

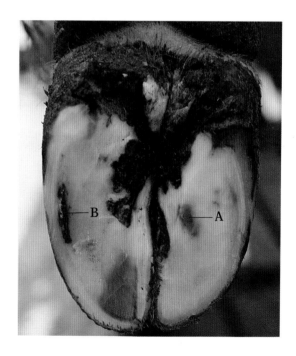

PLATE 2.6   A sole haemorrhage. Note blood at the sole ulcer site (A) and at the white line (B). The black at the toe is the normal hoof pigment.

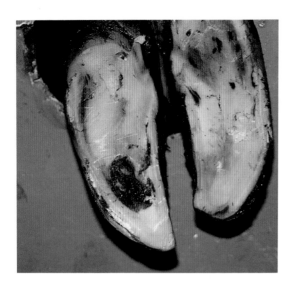

PLATE 2.7 A sole haemorrhage. Note blood at the toe and at the white line. The right claw has diffuse haemorrhage and yellow discolouration throughout.

Note the blood clots at the sole ulcer site and at the toe, these being the front and rear contact points of the pedal bone with the solar hoof beneath. Such areas are often referred to as 'bruising'. It is a type of bruising, but of course the bruise developed some 8–12 weeks ago (horn grows at 5mm per month and the sole is approximately 10–15mm thick) and has only just appeared at the surface.

In some cows, removing a few superficial slivers of horn removes the bloodstained area and leaves intact horn beneath. In this instance, bruising would have taken place over a very limited period of time. In other animals (and usually over the sole ulcer site), the mixture of blood and horn is continuous down to the corium, indicating that bruising is still occurring. Plate 2.7 shows severe haemorrhage at the toe.

Digital Cushion

Towards the heel the pedal bone is separated from the corium by the digital cushion, a pad of fibro-elastic tissue which acts as a shock absorber. As the foot makes contact with the ground there is an initial braking force exerted between the pedal bone and its suspensory laminae and then a slight movement of pedal bone at the heel, leading to compression of the digital cushion (58).

Tendons

Bending the leg forwards and backwards is achieved by tendons, one end of which is attached to a muscle and the other end to a bone. When the muscle contracts, it shortens and, via the tendon, pulls and moves the bone.

There are two major tendons in the foot: the extensor tendon, which extends the joints of the leg and helps to pull the leg forwards, and the flexor tendon, which pulls the leg back and flexes the foot.

As tendons are also involved in weightbearing and act as shock absorbers, they must be very strong. The thick, glistening white flexor tendon can be seen in Plate 2.2. It runs down the back of the leg in an enclosed lubricated sheath (the tendon sheath) and attaches to the rear edge and base of the pedal bone.

Navicular Bone

Where the tendon changes direction within the heel bulb, there is another small bone, the navicular (sometimes called the distal sesamoid) bone, which facilitates movement of the tendon. This is shown in Figure 2.11 and Plate 2.8.

Navicular Bursa

A lubricated area, the navicular bursa, which lies between the tendon and the bone, allows easy movement between the two structures. Note how the sole ulcer site is immediately below the point of insertion of the flexor tendon onto the pedal bone. If the ulcer penetrates deep into the corium, small white or creamy white strands of fibrous material are

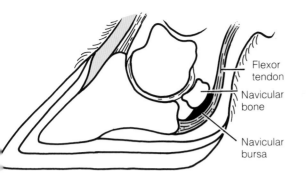

FIGURE 2.11   Position of the navicular bone, navicular bursa and flexor tendon.

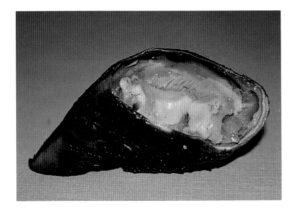

PLATE 2.8   A hoof showing the pedal bone and navicular bone in situ.

sometimes seen. These are fragments of the degenerating flexor tendon. Deeper penetration of infection from an ulcer can produce an abscess in the navicular bursa. Affected cows will have an enlarged, inflamed and very painful heel area, with reddening of the skin above (see Plate 5.26). Lameness will be intense. Often a small bead of pus can be seen discharging from the ulcer site, an indication that there is an abscess beneath with considerably more pus present.

The only treatment for such cases is drainage through a radical opening of the abscess (10). Advanced or untreated cases may lead to infection of the navicular bone, to infection penetrating the pedal joint, or even to degeneration of the pedal bone itself, when amputation of the digit may be necessary.

Pedal Joint

The pedal joint is the junction of the pedal bone and the second phalangeal bone.

The nomenclature of the bones and joints up to the fetlock is shown in Figure 2.12 and this can also be seen in Plate 2.2. Note how the rear edge of the navicular bursa and the front edge of the navicular bone are incorporated into the pedal joint. Infection in this area can cause serious damage and hence the importance of prompt attention to and treatment of lame animals.

HORN FORMATION AND LAMINITIS (CORIITIS)

As hoof overgrowth and many types of lameness are associated with laminitis, we need to understand exactly what laminitis is and what changes it produces, before progression to a discussion of its effects and causes.

Earlier in this chapter we saw how the stratum germinativum, the layer of cells of the epidermis covering the papillae, was the site of horn formation. By continuous multiplication, large squame (thin, plate-like) cells are slowly pushed away from the stratum germinativum. Keratin synthesised within their cytoplasm forms strengthening keratin fibres and as the cells shrink, dehydrate and die, they produce the very hard horn surface which we know as the outer wall of the hoof. Hoof horn consists of horn tubules (from the tips of the papillae) and intertubular horn (from the sides and crypts of the papillae) and both components consist of elongated squame cells filled with keratin. The more

13

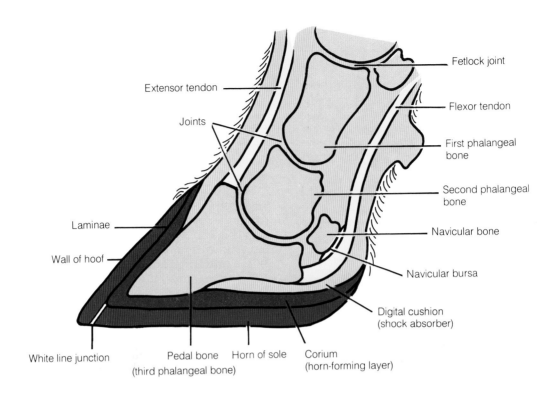

Fetlock joint

Extensor tendon

Joints

Flexor tendon

First phalangeal bone

Second phalangeal bone

Laminae

Navicular bone

Wall of hoof

Navicular bursa

Digital cushion (shock absorber)

White line junction

Pedal bone (third phalangeal bone)

Horn of sole

Corium (horn-forming layer)

FIGURE 2.12   The structure of the foot: bones and joints up to the fetlock.

detailed structure of the horn of the white line is described on pages 7 to 8. It consists of elongated, keratin-filled squame cells in the laminar horn leaflets, with much more rounded squame cells in the interdigitating horn produced by the terminal edge of the laminae (see Figures 2.7, 2.8 and 2.9). There are. no horn tubules in this area.

Laminitis simply means inflammation of the laminae, although in effect all areas of the corium may be congested and inflamed. The term 'laminitis' is often used (as in the following text) to include a generalised inflammation of the corium. Probably the terms coriitis or coriosis would be more appropriate. This section of the book describes only the changes associated with laminitis. Its causes and control are discussed in Chapter Six.

Increased blood flow through the corium means that horn is produced more rapidly. This can lead to overgrowth of the wall or sole and may also result in less mature and therefore softer and less durable horn reaching the wearing surfaces. These changes are particularly prominent in the white line area.

By taking slivers of horn and examining them under the very high magnification of an electron microscope, detailed changes in the white line of heifers before and after calving have been described (40). The elongated intact leaflet horn cells are shown in Figure 2.8 and the rounded interdigitating cells in Figure 2.9. Note how the cell junctions were firmly fixed together, giving strength to the horn. After calving, the horn began to degenerate in almost all the heifers. This was seen as a separation of the squame cells (Figure 2.13), the spaces between them becoming filled with red blood cells, bacteria and general amorphous debris.

14

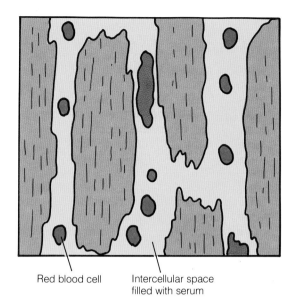

Red blood cell   Intercellular space
                  filled with serum

FIGURE 2.13   Section of white line in a heifer
after calving. The spaces between the squame
cells have enlarged and become filled with serum,
red blood cells, bacteria and general debris.
(D. Logue and S. Kempson)

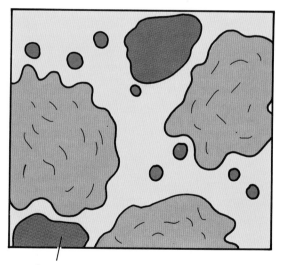

Degenerating squame cell

FIGURE 2.14   Advanced changes in white line
horn. The squame cells are degenerating, there is
little or no internal keratin, and the intercellular
spaces are large, filled with blood, serum and
accumulations of amorphous debris.
(D. Logue and S. Kempson)

The worst affected cells were very badly damaged. There were large spaces between them, cell membranes were disrupted and in some, keratinisation had been so badly disturbed that there was a complete absence of keratin fibres within the cell (Figure 2.14).

The net effect of these processes is a serious weakening of the structure of the white line, thus allowing impaction of debris or penetration of infection into the corium. The changes described are, of course, microscopic, requiring magnification of many thousands to appreciate their detail. On the hoof itself the same changes are seen as a yellow discolouration of the hoof or white line, as on the sole in Plate 2.7. This is thought to be due to blood vessels damaged by laminitis, allowing yellow serum to ooze into the spaces between the horn cells.

More severe vascular (blood vessel) damage can lead to the release of whole blood cells, again into the spaces between the squame cells, and this is seen as blood mixed with horn in the sole or white line area. Plates 2.6 and 2.7 are good examples. After calving, the cow in Plate 2.7 had its diet changed immediately from an all-forage precalving ration to a high fat, low forage, out-of-parlour ration (M/D = 11.7, where M/D equals metabolisable energy of the diet (Mj) divided by dry matter (kg)), plus 7kg of concentrates in the parlour, without any gradual introductory period of post-calving feeding. The resulting laminitis produced severe lameness, with haemorrhage at the toe, at the sole ulcer site and on the white line.

In some cases, congestion of blood vessels in the corium becomes so intense that blood flow almost stops. This results in reduced horn formation or, occasionally, complete but temporary cessation. Plate 5.48 shows a horizontal fissure running around the front of the hoof. This cow had been very ill with a coliform mastitis immediately after calving. Although she eventually recovered, the total interruption of horn

15

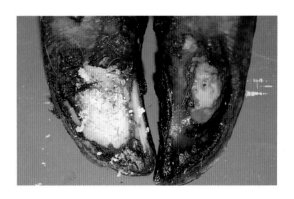

PLATE 2.9 *Pockets of soft powdery horn on the sole have been attributed to laminitis, but this material is normal sole horn which has not been worn away.*

formation, followed by resumption days or weeks later, led to two separate parts to the hoof. The lower 'thimble' should eventually have grown off the end of the toe (see page 57).

Less severe attacks of laminitis lead to grooves around the hoof, as seen in Plate 5.50. These have been referred to as 'hardship lines' (27). A series of parallel horizontal grooves indicates that the cow suffered repeated attacks of laminitis. The soft, powdery pockets of white horn, which may be found on the sole (Plate 2.9), are sometimes said to be a consequence of laminitis. This is not correct. The powdery material is simply old and degenerating superficial horn not removed by natural wear.

Figure 2.12 shows how the pedal bone fits tightly inside the hoof at the toe. Engorgement and enlargement of blood vessels in such a confined area leads to pain and discomfort. The affected cow tries to take the weight off her toes by walking on her heels and by turning her toes outwards. This decreases the height of the heel, makes the angle of the front wall more shallow and causes the cow to walk with her hocks closer together. These changes are shown in Figure 2.15 and in the stance of an affected cow in the frontispiece.

The longer-term effects of laminitis are eventually seen as an upward rotation of the toe and a convex shape of the anterior hoof wall (58), changes demonstrated in Figure 2.16 and in the affected foot shown in Plate 2.10.

So far we have looked primarily at the effects coriosis/laminitis has on the hoof. There are also dramatic effects on the suspension of the pedal bone within the hoof. As mentioned above, Figure 2.12 shows how the pedal bone fits tightly inside the hoof, especially at the toe. In fact the bone is suspended within the hoof by the laminae of the wall, with a much more effective suspension from the lateral (outer) wall than from the medial (inner) wall. If a heifer or cow develops a severe attack of laminitis, then this suspension breaks down and the bone 'sinks' within the hoof, dropping onto the corium of the sole. This can have several effects:

- if the rear end of the bone drops first, the corium becomes pinched at this point and a sole ulcer may be produced (see Figure 2.10 and Plate 2.6)
- if the front edge drops first, this will produce haemorrhage at the toe, as in Plate 2.7. This is sometimes known as a toe ulcer
- sinking of the pedal bone compresses and displaces the corium of the sole, as shown in Figure 2.17. If the corium is displaced to the side of the hoof, this will lead to an expanded and weakened white line, with an increased risk of white line abscess (Plate 5.1). If displaced upwards it produces a swelling around the top of the hoof, just above the coronary band. This is clearly seen in Plate 2.10

Once the pedal bone has sunk onto the corium of the sole, it will never regain its original position, and the affected animal will have to walk with a compressed corium for the remainder of its life. This can lead to permanent poor horn formation, particularly around the sole ulcer site, and in some cows the pedal bone will have dropped so much that its rear edge can be palpated just beneath the sole.

16

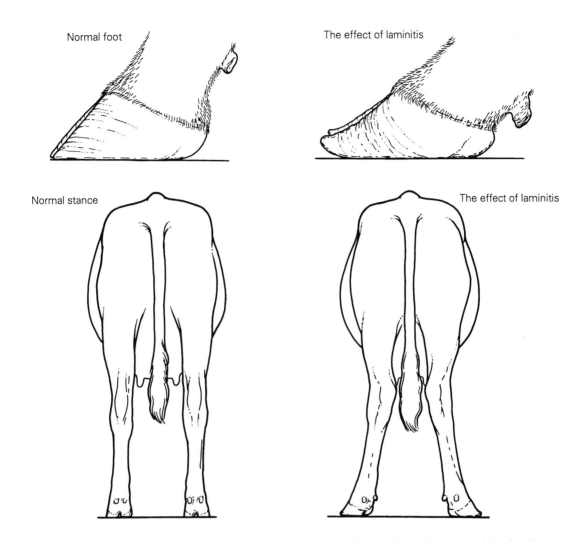

FIGURE 2.15   Changes in hoof shape and stance due to laminitis. The toe lifts off the ground, the heel drops and the angle of the front wall becomes much more shallow. Affected cows walk with hocks together and toes turned outwards.

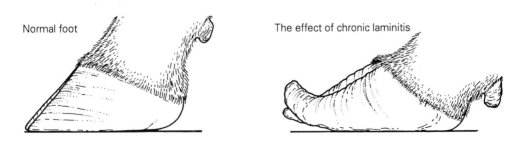

FIGURE 2.16   Chronic laminitis: a sunken heel, concave front wall and toe rotated upwards.

17

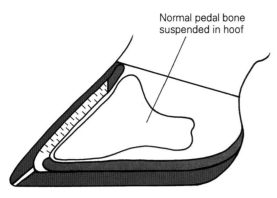

Normal pedal bone suspended in hoof

Displaced corium leads to swelling around coronary band

Laminae are disrupted, allowing pedal bone to sink in hoof

Displaced corium expands the white line

Pedal bone compresses corium at front and rear

FIGURE 2.17 Laminitis can disrupt the suspension of the pedal bone, allowing the bone to sink onto the corium of the sole. The corium may then become displaced laterally, leading to an enlarged white line, or upwards, producing swelling above the coronary band. *(Dr P. Ossent)*

In summary, therefore, generalised inflammation of the corium (coriosis), and this includes laminitis, may lead to any one of the following changes:

- pain and discomfort, especially at the toe, encouraging the cow to walk back on her heels
- upward rotation of the toe, a concave 'dishing' of the anterior (front) hoof wall and gross claw overgrowth
- hardship lines, which are horizontal grooves encircling the wall, or even a complete horizontal fissure
- yellow (serum) discolouration of the sole horn, with blood in the white line and sole ulcer site in more advanced cases
- sinking of the pedal bone, leading to displacement of the corium both to the side of the hoof (expanding and weakening the white line) and above the coronary band (producing a swelling above the hoof)

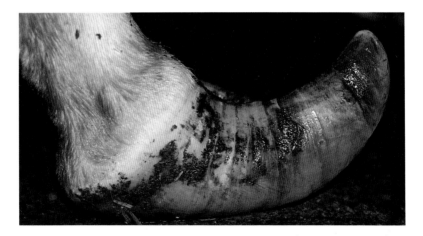

PLATE 2.10 *Chronic laminitis. Note the overgrown toe no longer makes contact with the ground during walking and the anterior wall is concave.*

18

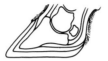 **CHAPTER THREE**

Weightbearing Surfaces and Hoof Overgrowth

The primary objective of hoof-trimming is to restore the foot to its correct shape and weightbearing surfaces. As such it is essential that there is first a thorough understanding of the normal foot and of the changes in hoof shape, structure and dimension which can occur with overgrowth.

WEIGHTBEARING SURFACES

In a correctly shaped hoof, weight is taken on the heel, on the wall and, to a lesser extent, on the white line area and 10–20mm of sole adjacent to it, running abaxially along the outside of the claw to the toe and then axially from the toe posteriorly along the first third of the interdigital space. This is shown in Figure 3.1 (*22, 28, 56, 58*). (If you are unsure of the terms being used, refer back to the explanations in Figure 2.1.)

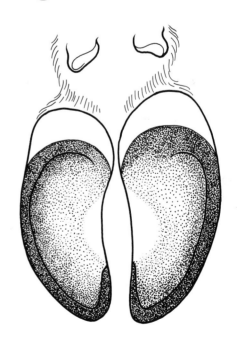

FIGURE 3.1 The weightbearing surfaces of the foot, indicated by shaded areas.

The whole area of the sole at the toe becomes weightbearing therefore, with weight being taken equally on the axial and abaxial walls. The unshaded area of sole on the diagram is non-weightbearing. The wall and sole should be flat from the heel to the toe, making even and consistent contact with the ground surface throughout and thereby maximising weightbearing. The inner and outer claws should be almost equal in weightbearing and the front angle of each claw should be quite steep, with the toe making firm contact with the ground during locomotion (*18, 58*). An axial view of a single claw, viewed from the interdigital space (Plate 3.1 and Figure 3.2), clearly shows how the wall runs posteriorly for the first third only (i.e. the weightbearing area) and then gradually merges with the sole.

The remainder of the axial surface of the claw, running back to the heel, consists of a concave area of sole (unshaded in Figure 3.1). This area should be kept clear and open and forms the interdigital space between the two claws. In a normal hind foot, **slightly** more weight is taken on the lateral rather than the medial claw. This difference is shown in Figure 3.1, where the medial claw axial wall particularly is smaller.

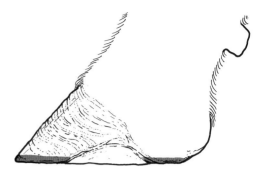

FIGURE 3.2 Axial (inner) view of a single claw, to show solar concavity, with weightbearing at the heel plus the first third of the axial wall.

Plate 3.2 shows a cross-section of two claws from a 14-month-old Friesian steer. Note how, even at this age, the lateral claw (left) has a significantly thicker sole than the medial claw. This difference becomes considerably more accentuated with overgrowth.

To optimise the efficiency of weightbearing within the foot, the anterior wall, from toe to coronary band, should be at an angle of 45 – 50 degrees with the horizontal, as in Plate 2.1. Provided that the anterior wall is straight, then of course the angle of the toe will be identical (45 – 50 degrees, see Figure 3.3).

The length of the anterior wall, often referred to as the toe length, or sometimes as the length of the dorsal border, should be 60 – 80mm, with the coronary band sloping slightly backwards, forming a shallow angle with the horizontal. This angle is, of course, determined by the height of the heel, which should be approximately 25 – 35mm for young cows and 30 – 45mm for older animals. However, these are average values only and, as one might expect, there is considerable variation in claw dimensions between animals (*4, 44, 51*). This variation is associated with factors such as:

- breed: Jerseys will obviously have smaller claws than Friesians or beef breeds

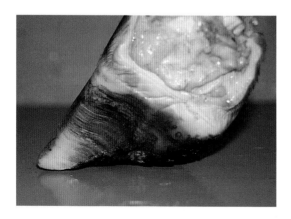

PLATE 3.1 Axial view of the claw, showing that weightbearing should be on the first third of the wall and heel only.

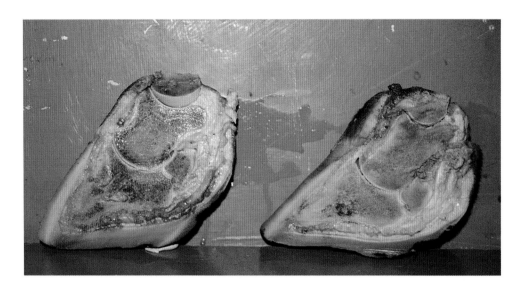

PLATE 3.2 *Sections of outer (lateral) and inner (medial) claws of a 14-month-old Friesian steer. Note the thicker sole on the lateral claw.*

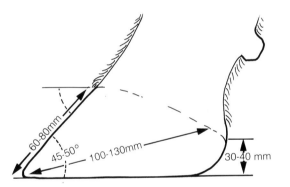

FIGURE 3.3 Approximate angles and dimensions of a normal claw.

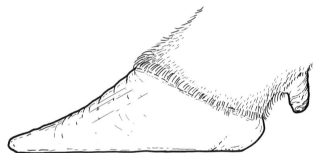

FIGURE 3.4 Cows with long toes and very shallow heels are best not retained for breeding.

- age: first lactation heifers have smaller claws than cows, adult size being reached by approximately the third lactation
- the differences between front and hind feet
- individual variation within a breed: some individual cows have abnormally large and/or shallow feet

Many hoof conformation factors have a high heritability; in other words they are highly likely to be passed on to the next generation. Cows with long claws and shallow heels for example, as in Figure 3.4, will produce offspring with similar defects. In the hind foot the angle of the toe has a particularly high heritability (4), so ideally you should not breed from cows with shallow hoof angles. It has been shown (51) that bulls with long toes and large soles are more

21

prone to sole ulcers than other bulls and this influence could be passed on to their progeny.

Conversely, foot-trimming, that is the restoration of the foot to a 'normal' shape, has been shown to improve the gait and locomotion score of cows quite quickly (*43*) (Table 6.4). When compared with untrimmed controls, the incidence of lameness also decreased. Hoof-trimming is therefore important, both economically and to the welfare of the cow.

As we have studied the dimensions of a normal foot, we can now examine where overgrowth occurs.

HOOF OVERGROWTH

There are three main areas of overgrowth, namely the toe, the lateral claw and particularly the sole of the lateral claw, leading to a disparity between the size of the two claws. Although all three occur simultaneously, it makes understanding easier if they are considered separately.

Overgrowth at the Toe

The shape of the hoof at any one time is a balance between the rate of growth and the rate of wear. The wall grows slightly more rapidly at the toe than at the heel, and hoof at the toe is much harder than at the heel. The net result therefore is that overgrowth occurs **primarily at the toe**. This has the effect of slowly reducing the angle of the toe from 45 to 40 to 35 degrees and the slope of the coronary band increases. These changes are shown in Figure 3.5.

In extreme cases of overgrowth (e.g. Figure 3.6), the anterior hoof wall becomes concave and the toe deviates upwards (Plate 2.11). Because there is then no longer contact between the toe and the ground, no wear occurs at the toe and overgrowth continues unchecked. Dishing of the anterior hoof wall is probably also an effect of laminitis (*58*). It

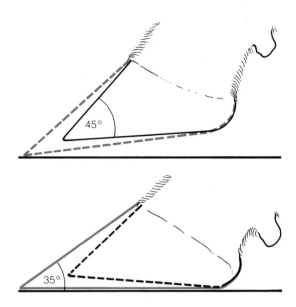

FIGURE 3.5   Hoof overgrowth occurs primarily at the toe.

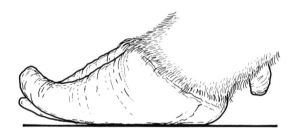

FIGURE 3.6   More advanced overgrowth, leading to a concave anterior wall and a toe which does not touch the ground.

is the wall that is primarily affected by overgrowth and hence there is often greater overgrowth on the abaxial (outer) side, than on the axial (inner) side of the foot. This is because the wall extends axially for only one-third of the distance along the interdigital cleft. The overall effect of this is often seen as a rolling of the wall under the sole, as demonstrated in Plates 3.3 and 3.4.

In addition to these external changes in hoof shape, there are dramatic changes

22

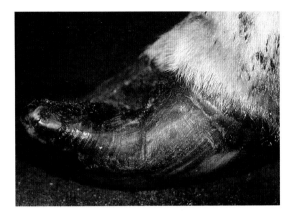

PLATE 3.3 An overgrown foot. Note how the toe no longer makes contact with the ground, the front wall is concave and the lateral wall rolls under the sole.

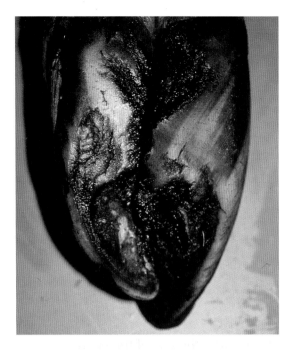

PLATE 3.4 Solar (plantar) view of the hoof seen in Plate 3.3. Note how the wall has extended across the sole to make the sole ulcer site a weightbearing area.

occurring within the hoof. Overgrowth at the toe leads to a backward rotation of the pedal bone towards the heel. Note the changing angle of the lower edge of the pedal bone in Figure 3.7. Plate 3.5 shows a cross-section of an overgrown foot with gross excess of horn at the toe. The foot has been tipped forward onto its toe for photographing, but when walking, this cow would be well back on her heels with the toe raised.

Erosion of the heel further exacerbates the backward rotation of the foot and pedal bone. Note how the posterior edge

of the pedal bone lies immediately above the edge of the eroded sole. The sole could bend at this point during weightbearing, further exacerbating the backward rotation of the pedal bone and discomfort within the foot, as seen in Plate 5.45. These changes are shown

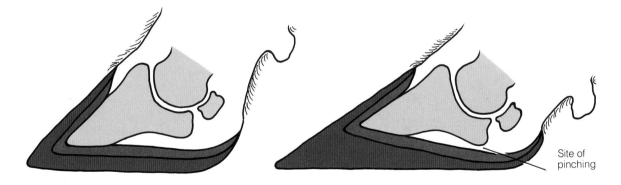

FIGURE 3.7 Overgrowth at the toe leads to a backward rotation of the pedal bone and pinching of the corium between the pedal bone and hoof.

23

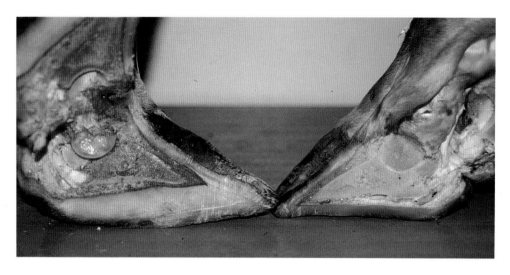

PLATE 3.5   A section of overgrown hoof (left) compared with a normal hoof (right). Note the excess horn at the toe and backward rotation of the pedal bone.

diagrammatically in Figure 3.8.

Although still suspended within the anterior hoof at the toe, the backward rotation of the pedal bone leads to more weight being taken along its posterior edge, i.e. towards the heel. During weightbearing and locomotion, this can produce a pinching of the corium between the pedal bone above and the sole of the hoof below, as shown in Figure 3.7. Pinching of sensitive tissues leads to pain; hence a cow walking on her

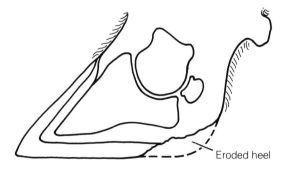

FIGURE 3.8   Erosion of the heel can further destabilise the foot. Note how the eroded heel may extend as far forwards as the rear edge of the pedal bone.

heels because of overgrown toes walks with considerable discomfort. We have all seen such animals, shuffling along with dropped pasterns and fetlocks close to the ground. The syndrome is less pronounced in the medial claw, because the pedal bone has a more effective suspension within the inner claw (58). Hence affected cows tend to walk by throwing their lateral claws outwards, trying to take weight off the lateral claw and transfer more weight onto the medial claw, as shown in Figures 2.15 and 3.9.

Pinching of the solar corium can lead to bleeding. Free blood is then mixed with horn as it is being produced, and moves down through the sole with natural growth, to be eventually seen as a small area of reddening, or maybe just a few red dots, in the solar horn at the typical ulcer site (see Plate 2.6). In fact it could be the start of a sole ulcer. This is dealt with in more detail on pages 45 to 48. The shape of the lower edge of the pedal bone makes the syndrome worse. Figures 2.3 and 3.7 and Plate 2.5 show that the pedal bone has a concave lower surface, leading to weight-bearing along the rear edge, i.e. exactly where the pinching of the corium occurs.

24

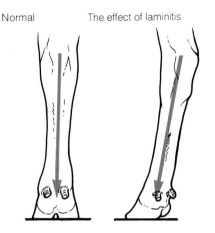

Normal   The effect of laminitis

FIGURE 3.9   Changes in hoof shape and stance due to chronic laminitis.

The importance of overgrowth at the toe has been demonstrated experimentally (56). Fixing a wedge to the sole at the toe increases the degree of flexion of the pedal joint. This in turn puts stress on the sole which becomes stretched, especially at the sole-heel junction immediately below the rear edge of the pedal bone. Within a few weeks the sole was found to be grossly thicker than the control claw and there were early changes indicating the start of the formation of a sole ulcer.

This is clear evidence of the importance of overgrown hooves in the formation of sole ulcers and of the fact that an overgrown toe leads to changes in the sole. Mild trauma may cause irritation of the sole corium and the production of sole overgrowth (Figure 3.12). More severe trauma and stretching may cause permanent damage to the corium and result in a sole ulcer (56).

By measuring the amount of weight taken on each claw during standing and locomotion, it has been cleverly demonstrated that there is a much greater **variation** in the amount of weight taken on the outer claw, compared to the weight variation on the inner claw (58). For example, when the cow is standing still and upright, weight is taken almost

evenly on both claws of both hind feet (Figure 3.10). As her weight is transferred onto the right leg, weight becomes increasingly distributed onto that leg, and particularly onto the outer claw, until the left leg is lifted off the ground. The same process then occurs when the left leg takes weight and the right leg is lifted off the ground.

It has been proposed that this great variability of weightbearing on the lateral (outer) claw leads to contusions (bruising) and exostoses (small bony growths) on the pedal bone of that claw similar to the changes seen in Plate 5.25 (58). These lesions lead to further pain, once again encouraging the cow to swing her legs out whilst walking and thus transfer more weight onto the medial (inner) claw. Both chronic low-grade inflammation of the foot and an abnormal gait can lead to

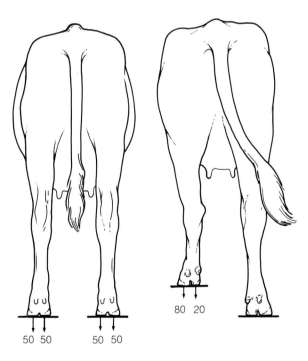

FIGURE 3.10   As the cow changes its weight from one foot to the other, there is a much greater variation in the weight taken on the outer claw than the variation in the weightbearing of the inner claw. This could be another reason why there is overgrowth of the outer claw on hind feet.

25

overgrowth of the lateral claw (a common feature in many dairy cows), thereby further destabilising the foot. This is demonstrated in Figure 3.11.

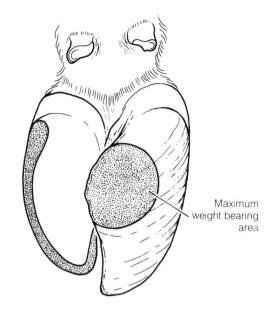

FIGURE 3.12   Overgrowth of solar horn is common on the lateral claws of hind feet. The shaded areas now become weightbearing (compare this with the correct weightbearing surfaces of Figure 3.1).

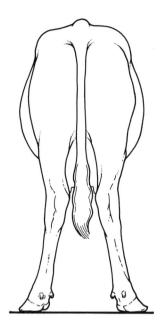

FIGURE 3.11   Overgrowth of the lateral claw of hind feet encourages cows to stand with their hocks together and throw their feet out when they walk.

Overgrowth of the Sole

Overgrowth of solar horn occurs on the lateral claw of hind feet and, to a lesser extent, on the medial claw of front feet. It is seen as a ledge of horn growing from the sole and protruding axially into the interdigital cleft (Figure 3.12 and Plate 3.6). The sole overgrowth may be so pronounced that it becomes the major weightbearing surface of the foot (Figure 3.12). This point is immediately below the posterior edge of the pedal bone of course, and further increases the chances of the corium being pinched during locomotion.

When the ledge is removed during hoof-trimming, there is often an area of pin-

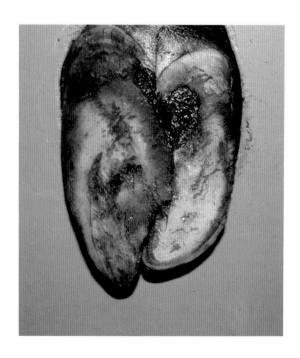

PLATE 3.6   *An overgrowth of solar horn.*

26

point bleeding or even frank haemorrhage into the horn at this point. It has been suggested that the various factors which lead to general overgrowth of the lateral claw also produce the overgrowth of the solar ledge. It is interesting that on front feet it is the **inner** claw which becomes larger and this is where the solar overgrowth occurs. It is also, unfortunately, the inner claw on front feet that most commonly develops sole ulcers.

Disparity of Claw Size

The third part of hoof overgrowth is seen as a disparity in hoof size. Several reasons have already been given for the fact that the lateral (outer) claws of hind feet become larger than the medial. For example:

- poorer suspension of the pedal bone within the hoof in the lateral, compared with the medial, claw leads to increased pinching of the corium
- a greater variation in load-bearing on the outer claw during walking
- a tendency for cows to stand with their hocks together and feet turned outwards, particularly following overgrowth at the toe

In addition, engorgement of the udder and metabolic changes leading to laminitis (coriitis) at the time of calving may also play a part. With an engorged and slightly painful udder, the peri-parturient cow will tend to walk by throwing her hind legs outwards in an arc-shaped swinging movement and she may stand with her legs slightly further apart. The outer claw would then make slightly less contact with the ground, would be worn less and hence overgrowth could occur.

By mid-lactation, when the udder has decreased in size, the lateral claws may already be overgrown and hence the cow continues to stand splay-legged.

It has been shown that haemorrhages and other changes in solar horn commonly occur at the time of calving, producing the subclinical laminitis syndrome (SLS) (27). (As there are no laminae on the sole, coriitis might be a more accurate term.) White line horn also shows degenerative changes following parturition (40).

The cumulative effects of all these processes could be to produce discomfort in the feet and hoof overgrowth, especially in the lateral hind claws. Foot-trimming aims to reverse these processes and is an attempt to compensate for the adverse effects of management, housing, feeding and breeding to which cows are subjected.

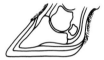

CHAPTER FOUR

Hoof-trimming

EQUIPMENT NEEDED

A variety of tools and equipment are available for hoof-trimming. The ones described in Plate 4.1 are those which I use. This does not mean that alternatives are not equally as good. Each individual must decide what suits him or her best.

A double-edged hoof knife is probably the most convenient to use. Alternatively have two knives, one for forward cutting and one for reverse. However, this entails changing knives each time a change in the direction of cutting is required and since I often do a few forward strokes followed by a few reverse strokes I find the procedure of changing knives exasperating.

Whatever the knife, it is important that it is **sharp**. A chain-saw file is small enough to get into the hook at the end of the knife and hence is very convenient. The sharpened knife can be protected during transit by wrapping it in a cloth, or inserting it into an old milking machine liner.

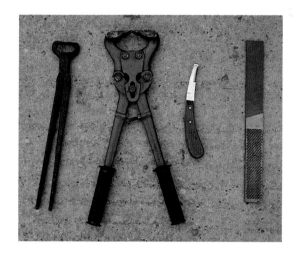

PLATE 4.1   Equipment for hoof-trimming: clippers, double-edged knife, file.

When hoof-trimming, and especially when searching the foot for pus tracks, it is best to cut with the flat blade of the knife, as shown in Plate 4.2. If only the curved tip is used, it is much more

28

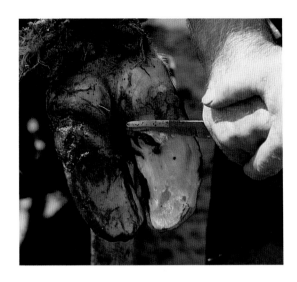

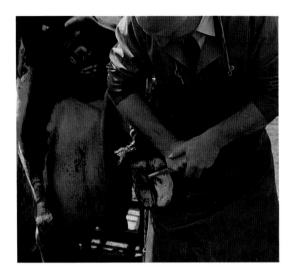

PLATE 4.2   Hold the knife with both hands and cut with the flat. Push down and across to give a sawing action.

PLATE 4.3   The position preferred for foot-trimming: behind the cow, facing backwards, with the cow's foot on the trimmer's knee.

difficult to identify lesions in the hoof and paring takes much longer. The knife should not simply be pushed vertically downward through the hoof. By moving the blade **across** the hoof (i.e. from left to right in Plate 4.2) at the same time as pushing towards the toe, a sawing action is achieved and this will make cutting very much easier. On a particularly hard foot (e.g. during a dry summer), keeping the blade wet also helps.

Personally, I find that standing behind the cow, facing backwards and sometimes with the foot resting on my knee, is the best position for trimming. This is shown in Plate 4.3. By holding the knife in both hands and pushing downwards to cut, much of the cutting force originates from the shoulders. In addition, it is a good position from which to visualise the claws and thereby achieve a balanced and correct weightbearing foot at the end of trimming. However, some operators prefer to stand facing the claw and cut by pulling the knife towards them.

A variety of clippers can be used for removing the horn from the toe (Plate 4.1). I use the type on the right in

the photograph, although the smaller ones on the left are much lighter in weight and have the advantage that they can be operated one-handed, the second hand then being used to position the claw.

Hoof shears are favoured by some as a method of removing large amounts of the hoof in one cut.

A surform or coarse file will assist with tidying the edges and sharp corners of the hoof when trimming has been completed. A file run over the bottom of the foot after trimming also makes sure that there is continual contact with the ground from heel to toe, thus maximising weightbearing. Similarly, the file can check that the axial and abaxial walls at the toe are correct and of equal height.

Protective gloves are a must if large numbers of feet are to be trimmed. They allow greater force to be applied to the knife and help to prevent the knife slipping when it gets wet or dirty. You only have to see how quickly a pair of cloth gloves wears through when foot-trimming, to realise how much damage must be being done to your hands!

On occasions I have used electrical grinding and cutting instruments, but have never found them particularly useful. Maybe I should have persevered for longer! A sharp knife with a good handle seems equally as rapid and effective and can be used to shape the foot. One possible danger of electrical devices is that unless they are used in skilled hands, excess hoof may be removed or the sole may be left excessively flat. In addition, some devices lead to overheating of the horn, with subsequent damage and hoof weakening.

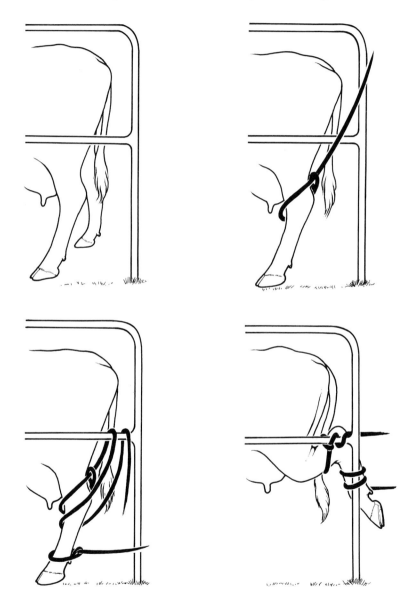

FIGURE 4.1 A system of using two ropes to lift the hind leg of a cow and tie the fetlock securely to the vertical bar at the rear of the crush.

RESTRAINT OF THE COW

Once again, this is very much a question of personal choice. Provided that the cow is restrained and supported so that she cannot struggle excessively or damage herself, and provided that the foot is sufficiently well restrained to avoid injury to the operator, but allows good, clear access for trimming, then the precise methods of restraint are not important.

Personally I do not favour roll-over tables. I find that the foot is not in the most accessible position for trimming and I do not like the way in which some cows slump to the ground when they are released from the crush. Belly-bands support the cow well, but they take time to apply and, in some cases, the cow hangs limp and has to be lowered to the floor before release. A single band placed immediately behind the front legs to support the chest provides excellent restraint when trimming front feet and with the band in position the cow will stand quietly.

Winches used to raise hind legs should have a secure self-locking mechanism and either a large wheel or a slow screw to turn for lifting. I have seen several frayed tempers and damaged hands when a struggling cow has inadvertently released a winch mechanism!

When using ropes I favour the system shown in Figure 4.1. A rope is placed just above the hock, using a slip-knot which tightens during lifting, thus discouraging struggling. The rope is wrapped round a side bar of the crush and back around the hock for a second time, before returning to the same side bar of the crush. This produces a 'pulley' mechanism. A second rope is attached around the fetlock. Pulling back on this second rope will make the cow kick slightly, thus lifting her leg. By pulling the first rope at the same time, the leg is lifted. The hock is secured to and level with the horizontal crush bar and the fetlock is fixed to the vertical. The cow is held firmly, thus reducing struggling, and yet she is well supported to reduce the chances of her falling in the crush. This system works best with two operators.

A similar system, but using one rope only, is the Pepper Footrope shown in Figures 4.2 to 4.5. It consists of a leg strap, and a supple rope with a shackle at one end, and a jamming cleat set into the rope a short distance from the shackle.

The ropes used should be moderately thick for both operator and cow comfort. If a winch is used, **make sure** that the metal clasp on the end of the rope does not cut into the cow's leg. (This happens all too often.) A short length of 2 inch wide belting, with a metal 'D' at each end, one larger than the other as shown in Figure 4.2, is ideal. The belt is placed around the hock, the small D slips through the larger D and the metal clasp is then clipped to the small D. A small loop of rope is a simple alternative to the belt.

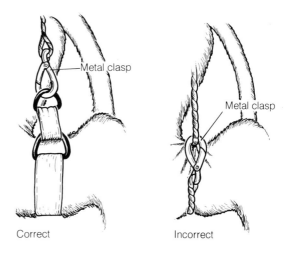

Correct   Incorrect

FIGURE 4.2   Do not use the metal clasp on the end of the lifting rope around the cow's hock. A strip of belting (*below*) or a short loop of rope provides much greater cow comfort and will encourage her to stand still.

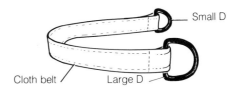

31

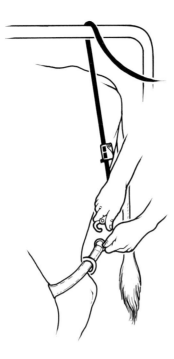

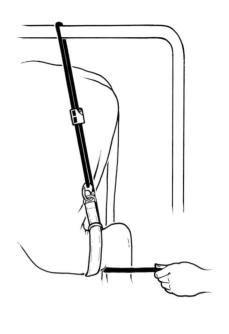

FIGURE 4.3   Secure the cow in a crush or standing, and lay the rope over the top bar or a beam. Place the leg strap around the hind leg, above the hock, by passing the smaller metal ring through the larger one. Attach the rope to the leg strap with the shackle. *(D. Pepper)*

FIGURE 4.5   Pass the rope around the inside of the leg, and tug sharply from behind, at a safe distance. When the cow kicks, keep the tension on the rope so that the leg is raised and held by the cleat in each new position. Having achieved the most comfortable height for the cow and operator, secure the leg to any convenient upright using the long end of the rope. *(D. Pepper)*

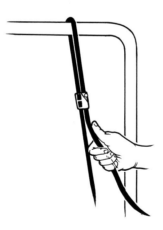

FIGURE 4.4   Thread the free end of the rope through the cleat, inside the guide, and down through the jamming part. Pulling gently downwards on the rope will take up the slack without putting any tension on the leg. *(D. Pepper)*

HOOF-TRIMMING TECHNIQUE

The objective of hoof-trimming is to restore the foot to its normal shape and weightbearing surfaces. In order to understand this procedure, it is important to read Chapters Two and Three first, which describe the normal hoof and hoof overgrowth.

There are essentially four stages of hoof-trimming. Although described as separate stages, in reality one stage merges with and constitutes part of the next stage, as the feet are slowly brought back into shape.

Cut One

Cut the overgrown toe back to its correct length, viz. approximately 75mm from

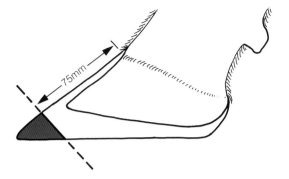

FIGURE 4.6   Cut One — cut the toe back to the correct length, approximately 75mm or one generous handspan.

Make the cut at right angles to the anterior wall, rather than at right angles to the sole, as this will reduce the amount of cutting required at Cut Two.

After Cut One, the foot is left with a square-ended toe, as shown in Plate 4.5. Compare this with Plate 4.4, which is the same claw before trimming. Plate 4.6 is a close-up of a cut toe. Note how at the toe the white line can no longer be seen on

the coronary band to the toe (Figure 4.6). This is approximately one hand-breadth. Place the thumb on the heel and the palm of the hand with the fingers not quite touching each other on the abaxial (outer) wall of the lateral claw. With the first finger just penetrating the top of the interdigital space, the toe should be cut off in line with the little finger. The width required is a good handspan, and be generous: i.e. leave slightly more rather than cut off too much. There is, of course, considerable variation in 'natural' claw shape (see pages 20 to 22). The distance described can only be approximate therefore and each cow must, to a certain extent, be assessed as an individual.

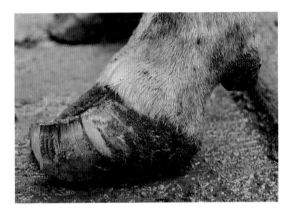

PLATE 4.5   A square-ended toe after Cut One.

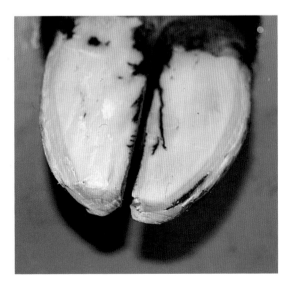

PLATE 4.6   The white line at the toe can no longer be seen on the surface of the sole, but it is visible across the cut end.

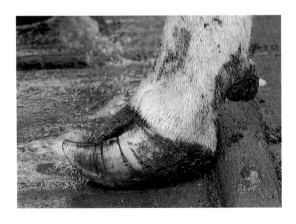

PLATE 4.4   A claw prior to trimming.

33

the sole, but is visible on the cut edge. Although the hoof is now the correct length, the toe is still too high (Plate 4.5) and the pedal bone remains rotated backwards towards the heel. Absence of the white line at the toe indicates that weight cannot be transmitted along the wall.

Cut Two

Draw a line from 'A', the top of Cut One, to 'B', the bottom of the heel and remove all the hoof from beneath this line, viz. remove the shaded area in Figure 4.7. Much of this will consist of removing horn from the toe. Provided that Cut One is in the correct position, there is no danger of penetrating the sole, although as trimming progresses the thickness of the sole should be repeatedly checked by applying pressure with the thumb in the toe area. As soon as any softening or 'give' is detected, further trimming must be discontinued. This can happen if Cut One is made too short, as demonstrated in Figure 4.8. Cut Two would now penetrate the sole.

Another common error is shown in Figure 4.9. Cut One is cut too short and to avoid penetrating the sole, the toe is left square-ended. This means that the wall at the toe is no longer a weightbearing

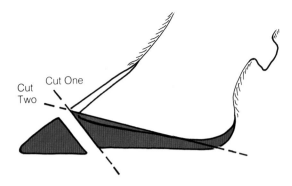

FIGURE 4.8   Cut One was made too short. Cut Two would now penetrate the quick (the corium) at the toe.

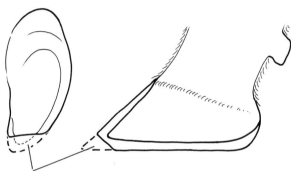

This section of the toe should be weightbearing

FIGURE 4.9   Cut One again too short and the toe is left square-ended. Weight cannot now be transmitted onto the wall at the toe.

surface and that it is the sole at this point which becomes weightbearing. This could lead to bruising of the sole and discomfort for the cow.

However, provided that Cut One is in the correct position, trimming off excess horn for Cut Two will slowly make the white line reappear, until it is once again visible running around the toe. This is shown in Plate 4.8 which is the same foot as in Plates 4.4 and 4.5, but with Cut Two completed.

This has the effect of bringing the wall of the hoof back up to a more upright angle and at the toe weightbearing has once again been transferred to the wall of

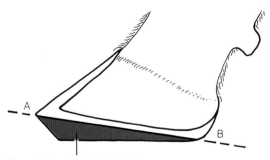

Repeatedly check the thickness of the sole in this area

FIGURE 4.7   Cut Two — remove excess horn, particularly from the toe, so that the anterior wall is brought back up towards the 45-degree angle.

34

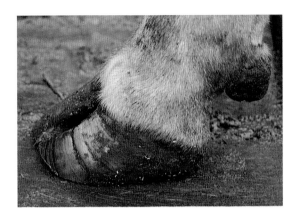

PLATE 4.7   Hoof-trimming complete. Note the
much steeper angle of the front wall of the hoof.
The toe is slightly off the ground, partly
because the cow is standing in the crush with
her leg forward.

the hoof. The front wall of the hoof has
returned to an angle much closer to 45
degrees and the pedal bone has been
tilted forwards, thus reducing possible
pinching action by its rear edge. In
Plate 4.8, which should be compared with

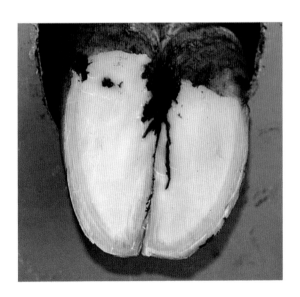

PLATE 4.8   Cut Two. By trimming excess sole
from the toe, the white line with the wall
outside slowly reappears.

Plate 4.6, the white line has reappeared at
the toe.
    Plates 4.9, 4.10 and 4.11 demonstrate
Cuts One and Two on a transverse section
of hoof. Note how in Plate 4.9 there is a
considerable overgrowth at the toe but the
heel is of normal height and this rotates
the pedal bone backwards.

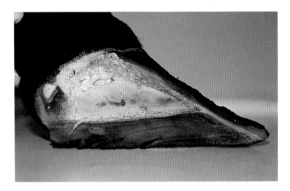

PLATE 4.9   An overgrown claw. Note the
excess horn at the toe.

    After Cut One (Plate 4.10) the wall and
white line at the toe no longer make
contact with the ground surface, i.e. they
are no longer weightbearing. Cut Two
returns the toe to a weightbearing
position and rotates the pedal bone

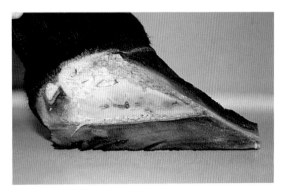

PLATE 4.10   An overgrown claw after Cut One.
The wall and white line area at the toe no
longer make contact with the ground.

35

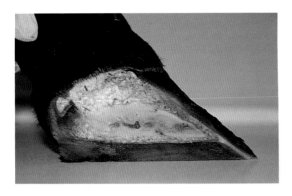

PLATE 4.11 The claw following Cut Two. Normal weightbearing surfaces have been restored.

forwards (Plate 4.11). The anterior wall of the hoof adopts a more acute angle. Some foot-trimmers leave a 5mm step at the toe when trimming cows prior to entering winter housing, thus allowing for growth at the toe. I can see no advantage in this.

Cut Three

Stage three consists of removing any ledge

of solar overgrowth from the lateral claw (or medial front claw), for example as seen in Plate 3.6, and 'dishing' the soles of both claws to produce a concave surface over the sole ulcer area (Figure 4.10) so that it does not bear weight.

This increases the space between the digits, making interdigital impaction by foreign bodies and dirt less likely and possibly reducing the incidence of foul and interdigital dermatitis. The additional space between the claws also reduces the pinching action on growths between the claws. Also known as interdigital fibromas, growths should be correctly called interdigital skin hyperplasia, since they are an overgrowth of skin. Increasing the space between the claws will often lead to their spontaneous resolution.

Dishing the hoof to produce a concave sole applies to the mid-third of the sole only. The axial wall ('C–D', Figure 4.10) running posteriorly for the first third of the distance from the toe must **not** be removed. It is an important weightbearing surface and should be at the same height as the adjacent abaxial wall.

When trimming is complete, points

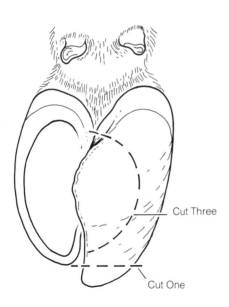

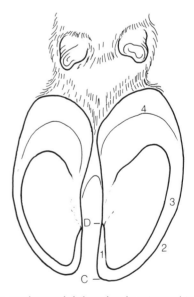

FIGURE 4.10 Cut Three — remove any overgrowth of the sole so that weightbearing is returned to the correct surfaces and specifically not on the sole ulcer area.

1,2,3 and 4 on Figure 4.10 should all be of equal height, that is, on the same level in a horizontal plane.

Removal of the axial wall is a common mistake made by many farmers and herdsmen. The theory that the toes should not be touching when trimming is complete is not correct. If the axial wall is removed, the claw becomes seriously destabilised, because it is only supported by one edge. Removal of excess axial wall can also lead to penetration of the corium at this point and, on more than one occasion, I have seen cows seriously lame because of over-zealous trimming in this area. Those unfortunate cases of white line abscesses and under-run sole which do involve the axial wall, almost always produce severe lameness and are slow to heal.

Cut Four

Overgrowth of the lateral hind claw, compared to the medial, is commonplace in dairy cows. The reasons are given on page 27. The fourth stage of hoof-trimming (Figure 4.11) consists of removing additional horn from the lateral claw so that it becomes equal in size to the medial claw. This effect can be best

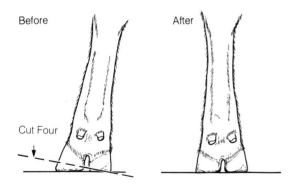

FIGURE 4.11 Cut Four — trim the outer and inner claws to an even size (left), thus bringing the legs and the stance of the cow back into an upright position (right). This normally involves trimming additional horn off the lateral claw in hind feet and the medial claw in front feet.

appreciated by referring to Figure 2.15 and by comparing Plates 4.4 and 4.7, which show a claw before and after trimming. Cut Four is one of the few occasions when heel horn has to be removed, but even then it should be done with caution and ensuring that an equal thickness of horn is removed from the heel to the toe. Removal of excessive heel horn could have the effect of tipping the anterior hoof wall away from the 45 degree angle, thus lifting the toe and rotating the pedal bone backwards to where pinching of the corium might occur. If there are loose flaps of badly under-run heel horn these may have to be removed however.

In a proportion of cows with severely overgrown and neglected claws it may not be possible to correct defects fully in one trimming session. This applies particularly to cases of laminitis where the anterior wall has become concave, as in Plate 2.11. Two or three attempts over a period of 9–18 months may be needed to restore chronically rotated digits to the correct stance and some will never fully recover.

GENERAL CONSIDERATIONS AND WHEN TO TRIM

Unfortunately, hoof-trimming is not a one-off task. Although trimming will undoubtedly improve foot conformation, gait and cow comfort, cows which walked badly before trimming will probably develop overgrown hooves again and will need further trimming. This is particularly so if some of the errors of management, feeding and housing discussed in Chapter Six are not rectified. Foot-care is therefore an on-going process, similar to measures a herdsman must take to control mastitis.

I believe that foot-care is the herdsman's task, and like many other tasks, refresher courses are beneficial and there are occasions when additional (veterinary) advice is needed. Routine foot-trimming has been shown to both decrease the incidence of lameness and improve the gait, locomotion score and therefore welfare of the cows (*18, 43*).

When is the best time to trim? Once again there are no set guidelines, but as a general rule feet should be examined:

- when lame or showing discomfort in walking
- when there is serious hoof overgrowth present. This is best detected as cows are walking through a herring-bone parlour, when both the sides of the hoof and the soles can be seen
- at drying-off. The advantages of lifting feet at this stage are that:
  - accumulated hoof overgrowth from the stresses of calving and lactation can be removed
  - as lameness is most frequent and has the greatest economic effect in early to mid lactation, feet need to be in ideal condition prior to calving
  - in occasional cows where trimming has been over-zealous, producing slightly soft soles, cows turned out to pasture at drying-off have ample time to recover

Perhaps at drying-off it would be better to think of **examination** of all feet rather than trimming. Many cows simply do not need to have the toe shortened, and just removing a few slivers of horn from the sole to check for impaction of the white line is all that is required. Dogmatic insistance that all toes must be clipped at drying-off is not only using unneccessary time, but it may also be deleterious to the cow in that either the toe is left 'square-ended' and does not bear weight correctly, or the sole is left excessively thin and soft.

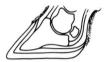

CHAPTER FIVE

Common Diseases of the Foot

Before discussing the various housing, nutritional and management factors associated with the prevention of lameness, it is clearly important to have some idea of the common diseases involved and their treatment. Some aspects of treatment can be carried out by trained farm staff, but other treatments need expert veterinary attention. Whenever in doubt, call for veterinary assistance. A cow is far too valuable to take chances with. In addition to welfare considerations, a wrong decision could result in much more expensive treatment later, or even the total loss of the cow.

WHITE LINE ABSCESS

The detailed structure of the white line and the effects of laminitis weakening that structure are discussed on pages 7 to 8 and 13 to15. Once weakened, small fragments of dirt, or even quite large stones, especially if they have sharp edges, can penetrate. The most common

points of entry are shown in Figure 5.1. Abaxially and towards the heel (site 1) is the most common, as this is the site

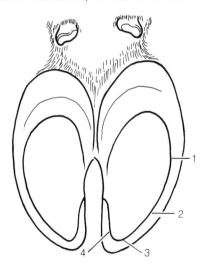

FIGURE 5.1   Common points of entry of infection in white line disease, given in increasing order of importance (1 to 4).

where, during locomotion, there are the greatest sheer forces between the rigid hoof wall, the suspended pedal bone and the movement of the heel contracting and expanding over the digital cushion. The severity of these forces is increased if there is overgrowth at the toe.

Following impaction of the white line with dirt, or penetration by stones, there are two possible scenarios. The continued growth of the hoof and white line may carry the debris to the surface, where it is worn away and eventually shed. Alternatively, further softening of the white line, or possibly standing on another stone, may force the material deeper into the hoof until it eventually reaches the corium (the quick). Such material will obviously be infected. The bacteria present will multiply, stimulating the defence mechanisms of the cow to produce pus. The pus accumulates, leading to increased pressure and this pressure produces pain and therefore lameness.

Although dirt may have tracked in through the white line, the hoof closes tightly around the track and it no longer remains a viable route for the pus to escape. As pus accumulates therefore, it spreads progressively between the corium (covered by epidermis) and the overlying hoof. This could be either under the sole (to produce an under-run sole) or under the wall.

Because the pedal bone is relatively tightly attached at the toe (Figure 2.3), there is less room for the pus to expand in this area. White line infection at the toe (site 3 on Figure 5.1), the axial wall (site 4) or at the first third of the abaxial wall (site 2) will cause a more acute lameness therefore. Site 4 can be particularly severe and slow to heal. However, there is more room for expansion towards the heel, and a white line infection at this point (site 1) may produce less lameness. In addition, the softer perioplic horn of the heel is more easily under-run and it is therefore easier for pus to track out and discharge at the heel.

Plate 5.1 shows typical lifting of the heel horn (A) where pus is escaping. The original point of white line penetration (B) can also be seen. Plate 5.2 shows the

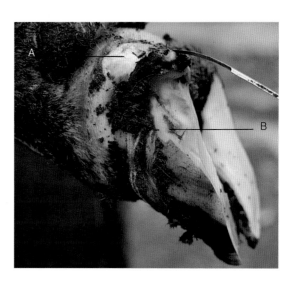

PLATE 5.1 *A white line abscess. Pus is breaking out through the softer perioplic horn at the heel at 'A'. 'B' is the original site of white line penetration.*

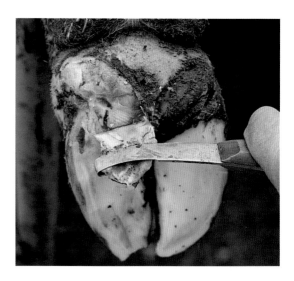

PLATE 5.2 *The extent of the under-run sole, all of which must be removed to promote healing.*

40

extent of the under-run horn, all of which must be removed if rapid healing is to be achieved. The pinkish-white tissue beneath the sole is corium covered by epidermis and this will form the new sole.

As soon as the pressure of pus has been relieved there is usually a rapid improvement in the severity of the lameness. Plate 5.3 shows a small bead of pus draining from another white line penetration site. Like any other abscess, the pus must be drained and hence all under-run horn is removed (Plate 5.4).

In neglected cases the corium may be so badly damaged that the pedal bone itself becomes exposed (Plate 5.5). Following

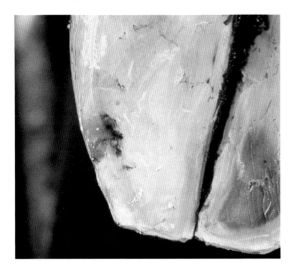

PLATE 5.3   Pus draining from a white line abscess.

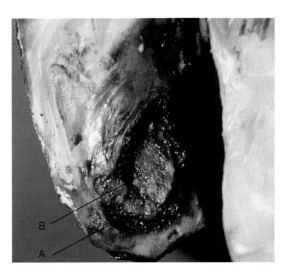

PLATE 5.5   In neglected cases the corium (A) may be totally eroded to expose the pedal bone (B).

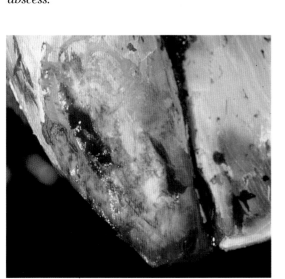

PLATE 5.4   Removal of under-run horn.

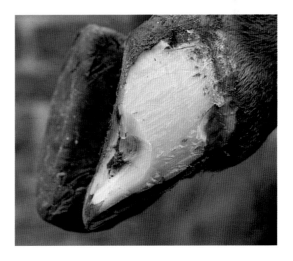

PLATE 5.6   White line infection discharging at the coronary band.

41

the application of a block to the sound claw, this cow recovered well and remained in the herd for at least a further three lactations. Plate 5.6 shows a white line infection which has tracked under the laminae of the wall to burst at the coronary band. Even in this case, all under-run horn has to be removed (Plate 5.7).

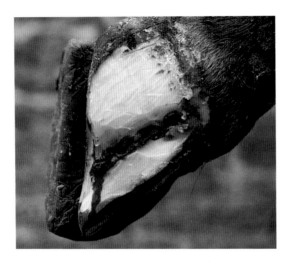

PLATE 5.7 *Track opened and drained by removing the wall.*

When draining a white line abscess, it is important that the small segment of wall adjacent to the infected track is opened up for drainage. If an attempt is made to drain infection by using only the curved tip of the hoof-knife, there is a danger that the hole will refill with dirt and debris and that lameness will recur. Removing a small segment of wall not only improves drainage considerably, but it also makes access to, and therefore removal of, further under-run sole or wall much easier. Plates 5.8 and 5.9 demonstrate this effect, but on a normal hoof.

The initial point of white line penetration may vary from a large, black area (Plate 5.10) impacted with obviously visible dirt, stones or grit, to a minute focus, no larger than a pinhead. When

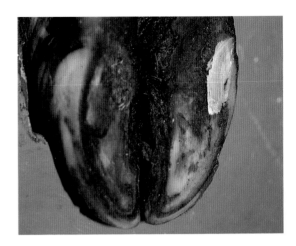

PLATE 5.8 *Searching for white line pus: a crevice cut out by the tip of the hoof-knife is likely to become impacted.*

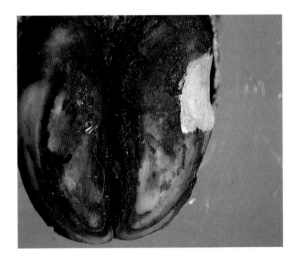

PLATE 5.9 *White line pus: removing the side of the wall prevents impaction of debris.*

some of these small tracks are followed down, there may be little more to see than a small change in the colouring of the horn.

As a general rule, if the track is black, it is going from the outside inwards, and should be followed. If it is red, for example as in the left claw of Plate 5.10, it

42

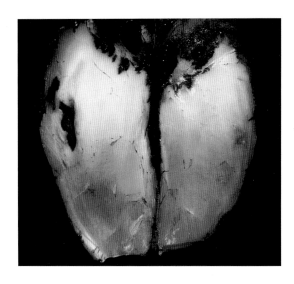

PLATE 5.10 *White line impaction. Note the large black track on the white line.*

is blood coming from the inside outwards, so it can be left alone. Large, homogenous black areas (for example, as in Plate 2.6 and in the right claw of Plates 5.3 and 5.4) should also be left. These are the normal black pigment of the hoof.

Opinions vary on the need to apply a dressing following removal of an under-run sole. An increasing number of people (including the author) consider that a dressing produces little additional benefit and if left on for long (i.e. more than a few days) it can be counter-productive.

There is no significant risk of infection from the environment penetrating this layer and, if left exposed, new horn forms very quickly. The application of a dressing, especially if it is bulky, both transfers the weight of the cow onto the corium of the exposed foot and retards drainage of infection and this, in addition to keeping the corium and hoof damp, may retard healing. At one time I almost always applied a bandage. I rarely do so now.

Fixing a wooden block or PVC shoe onto the sole of the sound claw, as in Plates 5.54 and 5.55, thus lifting the affected claw off the ground, is an

excellent treatment and rapidly facilitates healing. White line lesions in the axial wall (site 4 on Figure 5.1) are particularly painful and are strong candidates for such treatment. The technique is described on pages 59 to 61.

In a proportion of cases lameness appears to improve following drainage of pus, but then recurs 5 – 7 days later. Re-examination of the foot may reveal a dark black-red, fleshy lump of granulation tissue (proud flesh) pushing through the wound, as in Plate 5.11. There is also slight swelling and reddening of the hairless coronary area. This is usually an indication that further under-run horn exists.

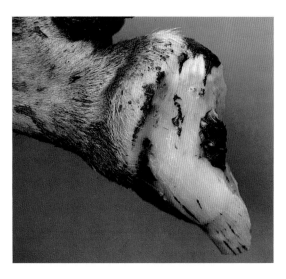

PLATE 5.11 *Protrusion of granulation tissue.*

In this case, the wall was under-run to the coronary band. Removal of the wall (Plate 5.12) and application of a wooden block to the sound claw effected a fairly rapid recovery. (Granulation tissue has no nerve supply and hence its removal causes little pain.)

In advanced or neglected cases, the affected claw starts to swell and may discharge at the coronary band (Plate 5.13). The cow will be acutely lame. This is an indication that infection has

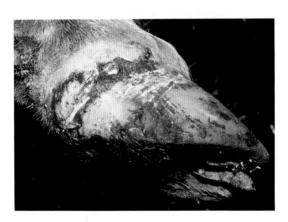

PLATE 5.12   Amputation of granulation tissue and removal of further under-run wall.

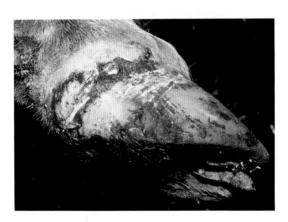

PLATE 5.13   Claw swollen at the coronary band with infection of deeper tissues. Radical treatment is required. (D. Weaver)

penetrated deeper structures, for example the navicular bursa, the navicular bone, flexor tendon sheath or even the pedal joint itself. (These structures are shown in Figure 2.12 and Plates 2.2 and 3.2.) Veterinary attention should be sought rapidly for such cases, as they will require drainage of the deep tissues and aggressive antibiotic therapy.

FOREIGN BODY PENETRATION OF THE SOLE

Although penetration of the white line is by far the most common site of penetration in the foot (because it is a point of weakness), any part of the sole can be damaged by a sharp object.

Typical foreign bodies are sharp stones, pieces of glass or tin, nails (especially those used for securing felt, which are short with a large flat head), and I have even seen the sharp roots of cast teeth penetrating the sole!

Sometimes, when a lame cow is examined, the foreign body is still present, but often it is missing and all that remains is a black track, distinguishable from a white line penetration lesion only by its position, viz. it is not on the white line (Plate 5.14).

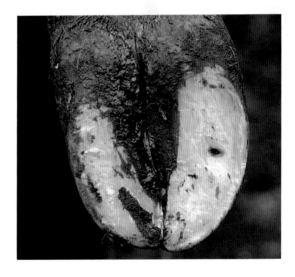

PLATE 5.14   Foreign body (nail) penetration of the sole.

It is not sufficient simply to remove the nail (or other foreign body) from the sole, since it will have carried infection in with it and the original point of entry will not provide sufficient drainage. The hole should be opened and all under-run sole

44

and adjacent wall removed (Plate 5.15). As with white line penetration, the lesion consists of separation of horn from the horn-forming tissue, so that when the under-run sole has been removed, new horn is exposed. The application of a dressing is therefore optional. Most cases probably heal better without one.

Plate 5.16 shows a stone impacted into the sole of a bull's foot. The cavity left in the sole after the stone has been removed (Plate 5.17) needs to be opened up by further paring, otherwise more debris might become impacted.

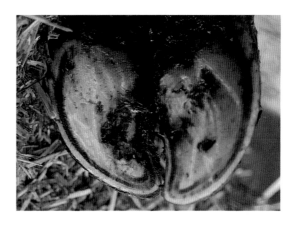

PLATE 5.17   The cavity left by the stone. This must be pared away.

SOLE ULCER

Sole ulcers typically occur on the lateral (outer) claw of the hind foot and, less commonly, on the medial (inner) claw of front feet and are characteristically sited in the central solar area, towards the heel. They are often covered by a ledge of solar horn, which protrudes towards the interdigital space. A typical ledge is seen in Plate 3.6. Sometimes the surface of the hoof appears normal; only when dishing the axial sole area during routine hoof-trimming (page 36) is the ulcer detected.

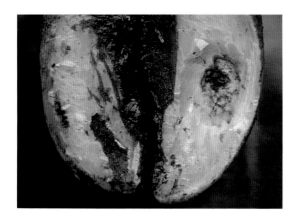

PLATE 5.15   Removal of under-run sole following nail penetration.

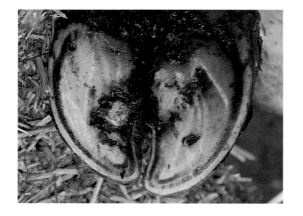

PLATE 5.16   A stone impacted into the sole of a bull's foot.

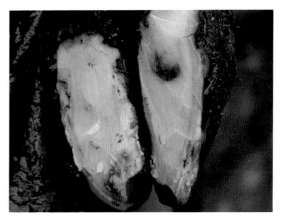

PLATE 5.18   Haemorrhage at the sole ulcer site.

Some appear as a central haemorrhagic area (Plate 5.18), which on further paring reveals an ulcer and under-run sole beneath (Plate 5.19). In others, such as the heifer depicted in Plates 5.20 to 5.22, the haemorrhage extends to the axial wall at the interdigital space. There is little to see superficially, but removal of a sliver of solar ledge reveals typical haemorrhage (Plate 5.20) which initially increases in severity with increasing depth. However, comparison of Plate 5.22 with Plate 5.21 shows how the haemorrhage is arranged in layers down through the sole.

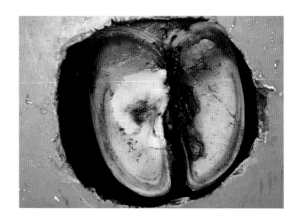

PLATE 5.20   *Haemorrhage in the sole of a heifer's foot.*

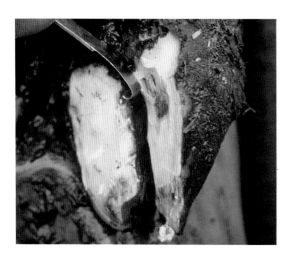

PLATE 5.19   *Ulcer and adjacent under-run sole.*

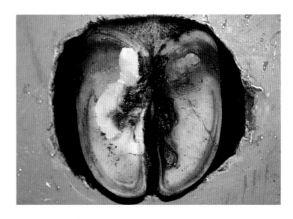

PLATE 5.21   *Exposure of the sole ulcer.*

The haemorrhage in Plate 5.21 could be trimmed away, leaving normal horn beneath. The distance from the solar corium to the most superficial haemorrhage gives an indication of when the initial laminitic insult, producing the sole ulcer, first occurred, since horn grows at approximately 5mm per month (see page 6).

The mechanics of the production of haemorrhage at this point are described in Chapter Two and the various management factors are discussed in Chapter Six. White line abscesses and penetration of the sole are caused by

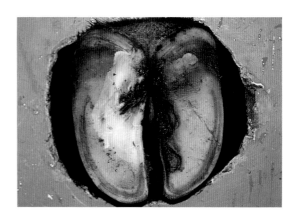

PLATE 5.22   *At this deeper level much of the haemorrhage in the sole has been pared away.*

external trauma to the sole and lead to separation of the horn from the horn-forming tissue.

On the other hand, a sole ulcer develops from changes within the foot and causes damage to the horn-forming tissue and the underlying corium itself. New horn is therefore much slower to form and a sole ulcer is much slower to heal. Many ulcers never fully recover and cows may remain with a chronic low-grade lameness, needing corrective foot-trimming 2 – 4 times a year for the rest of their productive lives.

Treatment consists of three main steps:

1. Dish the sole as much as possible, so that weight is no longer taken on the ulcer area. This was done for the heifer in Plates 5.20 to 5.22. Where possible, pare back the affected claw to its minimum size, but leave the sound claw large and weightbearing, thus taking further weight off the ulcer.
2. Remove infected and under-run horn from around the edge of the ulcer, viz. remove the horn being lifted by the hoof-knife in Plate 5.19.
3. Often lumps of granulation tissue

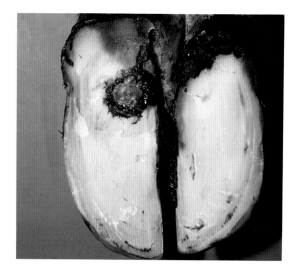

PLATE 5.23   *Proud flesh protruding from the ulcer.*

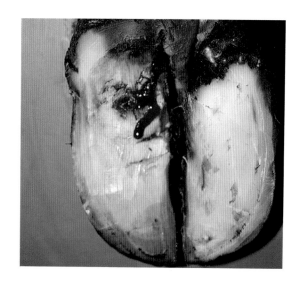

PLATE 5.24   *Proud flesh amputated.*

(proud flesh) protrude from the ulcer site, as in Plate 5.23. These should be amputated flush with the sole (Plate 5.24), thus allowing new horn to grow over the initial lesion.

The value of a copper sulphate dressing or other astringents, or even a calf disbudding iron to burn out granulation tissue within the ulcer, is debatable (*11*). While it might destroy the granulation tissue, I feel that it also damages the developing new horn (i.e. the corium and its covering of epidermis) and is therefore contra-indicated.

A bulky bandage retaining the dressing would transfer weight onto the ulcer site, thus increasing bruising of the area and retarding healing. However, others consider that a dressing is worthwhile. As ulcers are slow to heal, glueing or nailing a block onto the sound claw, to remove weightbearing from the ulcer, is an excellent measure to promote healing.

Ulcers are situated on the sole of the foot, just beneath the posterior tip of the pedal bone, at the point of attachment of the deep flexor tendon (Figure 2.10 and Plate 5.45). In Plate 5.45 note how the horn of the sole has become indented by

47

the rear edge of the pedal bone at 'A', and how loss of the heel at 'B' further destabilises the foot.

Plate 5.25 compares a normal pedal bone (right) with a boiled-out specimen from a cow with a chronic and long-standing sole ulcer (left). Note how the base and edges of the affected bone are roughened with exostoses (bony overgrowths), especially around the joint. This will lead to pain and discomfort when walking. As the exostoses will persist even when the ulcer has healed, early detection and prompt and effective treatment is important if such permanent damage is to be avoided.

Penetrating infection from a deep ulcer could lead to abscess formation in the digital cushion, the navicular bursa, navicular bone or even the pedal joint itself.

When deeper infections are involved, there will be swelling of the skin above the coronary band and application of pressure to the heel may produce a purulent discharge from the original ulcer site. Pus can be seen discharging from an ulcer in Plate 5.26. A wooden block has been applied to the sound claw. Such cows will be acutely lame and veterinary attention is needed to produce drainage of infection from these deeper tissues. Total rupture of the deep flexor tendon may occur, leaving the cow with a permanently turned up toe, as seen in Plate 5.27.

SOLE HAEMORRHAGE

Haemorrhagic areas, combined with softening and/or yellow discolouration of the horn, may occur in other parts of the sole in addition to the sole ulcer site and either with or without an ulcer. These changes are associated with an increased frequency of other diseases of the digit and have been termed the subclinical laminitis syndrome, SLS (27). However, some researchers (56) who have carried out a detailed microscopic examination of these changes state that although there is loss of onychogenic substance (i.e. horn-forming tissue) laminitis is not involved. Presumably this is simply because the haemorrhage occurs in areas of the sole where there are no laminae.

A variety of possible causes for the discolouration and haemorrhage in the sole have been suggested, with high starch and other carbohydrate-rich diets being the most important. Other factors include excessively rapid growth (and therefore high concentrate diets) during rearing; sudden changes in diet, especially from low to high concentrate rations; rapid changes in the amount of exercise;

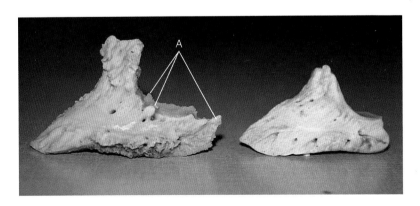

PLATE 5.25   A long-standing sole ulcer leads to irreversible changes in the pedal bone. A normal bone is shown on the right. Note the exostoses (A) on the left pedal bone.

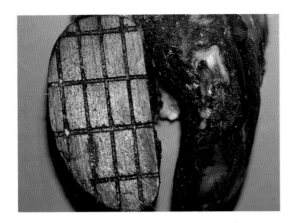

PLATE 5.26 *Pus oozing from the sole ulcer, an indication that deeper structures are involved and more radical treatment is needed.*

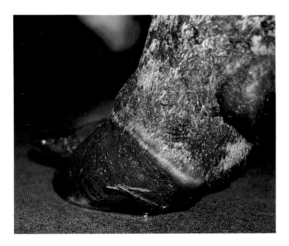

PLATE 5.27 *Dorsal (upward) rotation of the toe following rupture of the deep flexor tendon.*

sudden movements (for example, when recently introduced heifers first encounter, and have to escape from, adult cows higher in the pecking order); excessively wet feet; and breeding and genetics. A sudden and abrupt change from a soft floor surface (e.g. pasture) onto hard concrete will also increase the incidence of laminitis, coriitis and sole haemorrhage. Heifers introduced into the herd in the summer (when cows are still outside grazing) are less likely to develop severe lameness than those introduced directly into full winter housing. This will be particularly important if there has been no prior cubicle training.

Plates 2.6 and 2.7 show acute sole haemorrhage, plus a sole ulcer, from a cow in a herd which was experiencing a serious lameness problem. The blood clot at the toe in Plate 2.7 probably resulted from intense congestion and swelling of the laminae in the restricted space of the toe, forcing the anterior (front) tip of the pedal bone downwards, thus pinching the corium between the pedal bone and the solar hoof and causing bleeding. This two-year-old heifer had calved two months previously and the laminitis was probably the result of a sudden change from a high fibre to a high concentrate ration, combined with excessive standing in wet conditions (i.e. a reluctance to use the cubicles) and the need to make sudden, pivoting movements in order to escape from older cows. When re-examined 4–6 weeks later, ulcers were found on both hind claws causing her to walk stiffly. By this stage it is likely that the pedal bones had dropped within the hoof and were compressing the corium of the sole (see Figure 2.17).

Haemorrhages at the toe are also seen occasionally in the front feet of working bulls, presumably due to trauma when dismounting from oestrus cows.

INTERDIGITAL CORNS OR GROWTHS
(INTERDIGITAL SKIN HYPERPLASIA)

These are also called interdigital granulomas, tylomas or fibromas, but the correct name is interdigital skin hyperplasia, since the lump is simply an overgrowth of normal skin. A typical example is seen in Plate 5.28. In every cow there is a small fold of skin adjacent to the axial (inner) wall of each claw in the interdigital space and hence hyperplasia can develop from either side. Chronic irritation to the underlying skin,

49

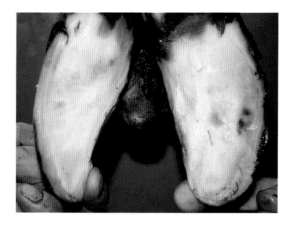

PLATE 5.28   Interdigital skin hyperplasia.

for example due to impaction of dirt or
low-grade interdigital infections, has been
suggested as one cause. In other cases the
condition may be inherited, being seen
particularly in heavy breeds of dairy cows
and in certain beef bulls (e.g. Herefords).
Lameness is due to the claws compressing
and pinching the swelling during
walking.

Secondary infection may occur,
producing foul (Plate 5.29), or an

inflamed area of interdigital dermatitis
may be found on the top of the skin
hyperplasia (Plate 5.30). Both conditions
need specific treatment.

Simply removing horn from between
the claws, thereby increasing the space
within the interdigital cleft, is sufficient
treatment for small skin hyperplasia

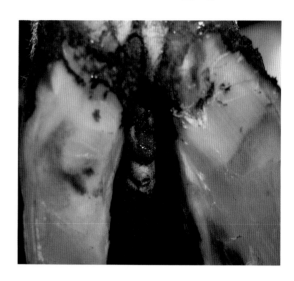

PLATE 5.30   Interdigital skin hyperplasia with
secondary interdigital dermatitis.

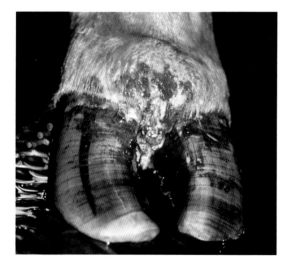

PLATE 5.29   Interdigital skin hyperplasia with
secondary foul.

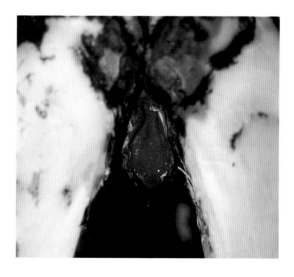

PLATE 5.31   Large interdigital skin
hyperplasia lesions require amputation.

lesions. If it is no longer being pinched between the claws, the skin hyperplasia slowly disappears. Larger lesions require veterinary amputation, as shown in Plate 5.31.

FOUL IN THE FOOT

This is also known (incorrectly) as foot rot and there are a variety of colloquial names such as 'lewer' and 'claw ill'. The correct name for the condition is interdigital necrobacillosis. It is caused by an infection with the bacterium *Fusobacterium necrophorum*, possibly in association with a second bacterium, *Bacteroides melaninogenicus*. Damage to the interdigital skin, either by stones, sticks or spirochaete bacteria, is thought to be needed before *Fusobacterium* can penetrate the underlying tissues.

Initially seen as a swelling of the coronary band (e.g. in the heifer in Plate 5.32), which forces the two claws slightly apart, the characteristic feature of foul is a split in the interdigital skin, often discharging pus and lumps of degenerating tissue debris, as in Plate 5.33. Some say that there is a characteristic smell. Personally I am not convinced about this. The important feature in diagnosis is that the interdigital skin is split.

In untreated cases the swelling may track up the leg towards the fetlock. In Plate 5.33 the deep interdigital erosion caused by foul is also penetrating under the sole of the left claw and must be extremely close to the pedal joint at this point.

Treatment, which should be administered promptly in order to avoid infection penetrating the joint, is normally by antibiotic injection. Also the foot should always be lifted to ensure that there is not a stick or stone between the claws contributing to the foul.

Formalin foot-baths (see page 76) are very effective in the control of herd outbreaks. If a high incidence of infection occurs, check that the feet are not being damaged by stones etc, for example in muddy and poorly maintained gateways. Outbreaks of foul can also occur in youngstock, both housed and at pasture. Individual cases may be seen in quite young calves, e.g. 2 – 3 weeks old.

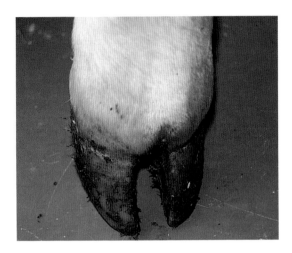

PLATE 5.32   A heifer with foul. Note the swelling of the coronary band and the claws forced apart.

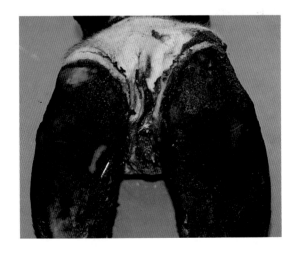

PLATE 5.33   Foul, showing the typical split in the interdigital skin exposing the underlying dermis.

DIGITAL DERMATITIS

First reported in Italy in 1972, digital dermatitis has spread across Europe to become one of the most common causes of lameness in the UK today.

Some texts refer to digital and interdigital dermatitis as two separate conditions, but as they are visually so similar and as both respond to the same treatment, it is highly probable that they are identical (*45*). Dutch authors (*58*) refer to heel necrosis (also known as slurry heel or heel erosion) as interdigital dermatitis. This terminology is not used in the UK or the US.

The typical lesion is first seen as a moist, light grey-brown, exuding area (Plate 5.34), with matted superficial hairs, situated on the skin at the back of the foot, just between the bulbs of the heels. There is a characteristic foul odour. Cleaning the surface exposes an irregular circular area, covered with diphtheritic debris (Plate 5.35) and red raw granulation tissue beneath (Plate 5.36). The lesion is intensely painful to the touch, surprisingly so, considering that it is restricted to the skin and produces no swelling of the associated tissues. In this respect it differs from foul, which typically produces swelling of the coronet extending towards

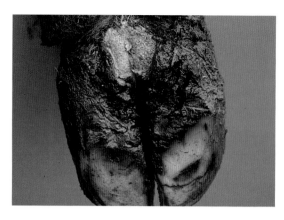

PLATE 5.35 Digital dermatitis: initial cleaning to reveal diphtheritic material.

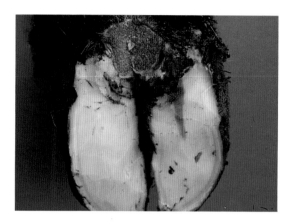

PLATE 5.36 Digital dermatitis: full cleaning reveals red raw and extremely painful granulation tissue.

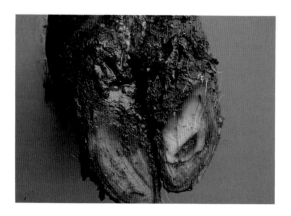

PLATE 5.34 Digital dermatitis: moist exudative area with matted hair.

the fetlock. Occasionally advanced lesions may develop hair-like filaments, as in Plate 5.37. In North America these are known as 'hairy warts'. Neglected lesions may erode the horn of the heel, producing an under-run heel (Plate 5.38).

The characteristic red, inflamed areas may also be seen between the claws (Plate 5.39), where it is sometimes termed interdigital dermatitis, on the surface of interdigital hyperplasia swellings (Plate 5.30) and, less commonly, at the front of the foot (Plate 5.40). At this site,

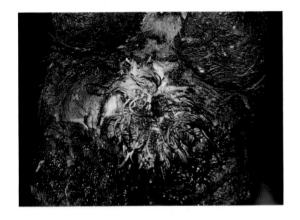

PLATE 5.37   Digital dermatitis: papilliform changes.

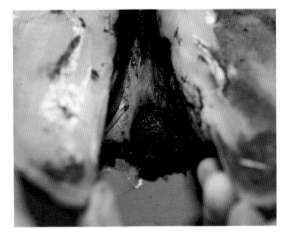

PLATE 5.39   Interdigital dermatitis.

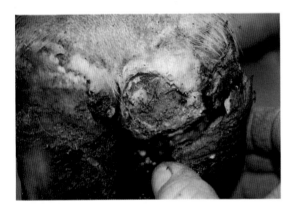

PLATE 5.38   Digital dermatitis and associated under-run heel.

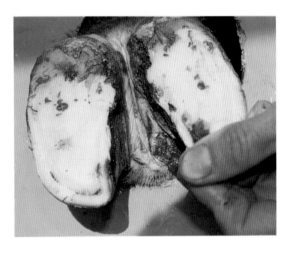

PLATE 5.40   Digital dermatitis: eroding the perioplic horn at the front of the foot.

erosion of the perioplic horn of the coronary band by digital dermatitis produces a much more severe and protracted lameness, involving underrunning of the front wall of the hoof. The deep infected cracks which occur on the axial wall of the hoof, and which are so difficult to trim, may be caused by digital dermatitis lesions which originate on the axial coronary band. Occasionally herd outbreaks occur, producing protracted lameness, often with a prolapse of proud flesh through the infected fissure (see Plate 5.47).

The precise cause of digital dermatitis is unknown, but the very prompt response to topical antibiotics indicates that a bacterial infection is likely, and an invasive *Treponema* spirochaete (*14, 52*) has been implicated.

Treatment is generally easy: simply clean the affected area and apply an antibiotic aerosol. Despite quite severe lameness, one treatment is usually sufficient. The exception is the lesion at the front of the foot. If the horn-forming tissue of the coronary band is involved, then a vertical fissure (Plate 5.47) may develop. Dermatitis at this site is hence best treated immediately with topical and injectable antibiotic.

Although individual cases of digital dermatitis do occur when out at grass, most herd outbreaks are in housed cattle and are associated with suboptimal hygiene (e.g. areas where stale slurry accumulates due to infrequent scraping), high stocking densities, insufficient cubicles for the number of cows and large herds. Immunity must develop following exposure because in established herds the disease is most commonly seen in purchased animals, or in recently introduced heifers, 2–8 weeks after entry into the herd (8). High culling rates and frequent purchase of new stock from a variety of sources probably perpetuate infection in an individual herd.

Herd outbreaks can be controlled by the use of foot-baths which contain an antibiotic solution. Formalin seems to have limited effects, if any, in the prevention of digital dermatitis. The antibiotic originally used was 2–4 g/l oxytetracycline for two or three consecutive milkings. Others have used a single bath containing 6–8 g/l oxytetracycline. Lincospectin is also effective. A 150 g pot containing 33 g lincomycin plus 66 g spectinomycin is sufficient for 200 litres of foot-bath at treatment level or 400 litres for prevention. Alternatively use lincomycin at 400 mg per litre.

The best response is obtained by walking cows into a herring-bone parlour and spraying their feet (and especially their heels) with a pressure hose (Plate 5.41). Allow to drain while the other side of the parlour is being filled, before walking the cows through the foot-bath. This takes a surprisingly short time, usually one bath is sufficient and it does not interfere with milking. The response can be dramatic. I have known several instances where the number of sorefooted cows declined markedly within 24 hours after the foot-bath and they stood more quietly in the parlour to be milked.

The cow depicted in Plates 5.34 to 5.36

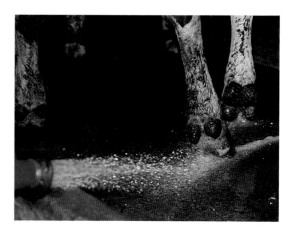

PLATE 5.41 *Digital dermatitis: spray heels with the pressure hose in the parlour prior to an antibiotic foot-bath.*

came from a herd where some 50–60% of cows were sore-footed or lame due to digital dermatitis. Careful hoof washing, followed by a single passage through an 8 g/l oxytetracycline foot-bath, produced almost immediate recovery.

MUD FEVER

Mud fever occurs following exposure to cold, wet and muddy conditions. One or more legs may be affected, the first signs being a swelling extending from the top of the hoof to above the fetlock. The skin becomes thickened and the hair encrusted. Hair loss occurs later, exposing the underlying skin, as in Plate 5.42. In more advanced cases the skin may crack to produce a raw, bleeding area, as seen in Plate 5.43. Lameness is not severe, especially if more than one foot is involved. Affected cows may stand and shake their feet, suggesting that mud fever causes irritation or severe itching.

For treatment, if possible house the cows or at least move them to dry conditions, wash any caked mud from their legs and, when dry, apply a greasy antiseptic ointment. Teat dips or sprays containing a high level of emollient are

54

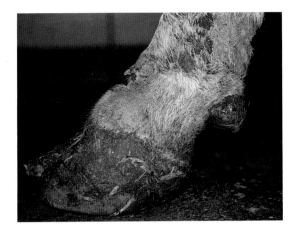

PLATE 5.42   *Mud fever lesions extending up the leg.*

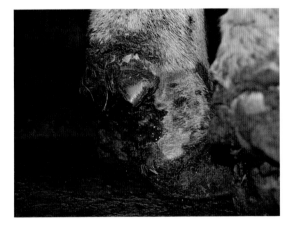

PLATE 5.43   *Mud fever: cracked heels.*

useful. As infection with the organism *Dermatophilus* may be involved, a three-day course of injectable antibiotic (e.g. penicillin and streptomycin) may also be beneficial.

HEEL EROSION OR SLURRY HEEL

The importance of an intact heel of the correct height for weightbearing and to maintain the stability of the foot is described in Chapter Three. In housed dairy cows, which stand for long periods in wet, corrosive slurry, the normal smooth intact horn of the heel becomes eroded and pitted and may become totally worn away. Plate 5.44 shows early heel erosion, whereas the cow with digital dermatitis in Plate 5.35 is quite badly affected.

The overall effect of this is to rotate the hoof backwards. The fetlock drops, the front wall of the hoof forms a much more shallow angle with the horizontal (i.e. decreases from the correct 45 degrees) and the toe may lift from the ground and no longer be weightbearing.

Internally, the pedal bone rotates back towards the heel, and may pinch the solar corium between its rear edge and the hoof, with resulting pain, lameness and possibly sole ulcer formation.

Although some hoof-trimmers remove the cracks and fissures in the heel, because of its extreme importance in weightbearing, I only pare the heel if it is seriously under-run, or if the heel is so badly eroded that the rear edge of the pedal bone is likely to be directly above the residual ledge of heel horn, as in Plate 5.45. Note how the horn of the sole has become indented by the pedal bone at 'A', and how the extensively eroded heel is missing at 'B'.

Regular formalin foot-baths reduce heel erosion, and attention to the environment, particularly removing

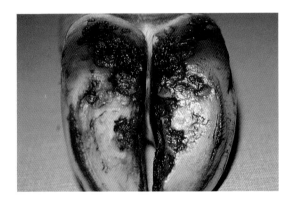

PLATE 5.44   *Early heel necrosis.*

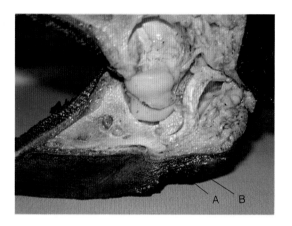

PLATE 5.45 *Extensive heel necrosis (B) has removed support from beneath the rear edge of the pedal bone, leading to sole indentation (A) and the start of the formation of an ulcer.*

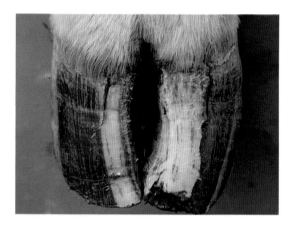

PLATE 5.46 *A vertical fissure (sandcrack).*

slurry and keeping the feet dry, helps to prevent heel necrosis. It is probable that the sprinkling of lime in the cubicles to reduce mastitis incidence also decreases heel erosion. A period of summer grazing is ideal, allowing the heel to recover and form again, ready for the onslaught of the next winter housing period.

VERTICAL FISSURE OR SANDCRACK

Sandcracks occur as a result of damage to the periople, the area of soft horn which originates at the skin–hoof junction at the coronary band. The periople gives a thin, shiny, wax-like coating to the hoof and covers the heel. Sandcracks are seen in older cows in hot, dry, sandy conditions and may also be secondary to digital dermatitis involving the coronary band. The damaged coronary area fails to produce intact horn and as the adjacent hoof continues to grow down over the laminae of the wall, the defect appears as a fissure in the wall.

Plate 5.46 shows a sandcrack in both claws, one extending almost to the toe. If it is shallow (viz. the laminae are not involved), no lameness results. However, because there is very little space between

the hoof and the pedal bone at the front of the foot (Figure 2.3), when infection occurs, just a minute quantity of pus is sufficient to cause severe lameness. Opening the track and draining the pus, using the curved tip of the hoof-knife, produces rapid relief.

If movement occurs between the two sides of the fissure, granulation tissue (proud flesh) may develop (Plate 5.47). This is best treated by removing the granulation tissue, opening the track slightly and, in severe cases, applying a wooden or rubber block to the sound claw, so that further movement within the fissure is limited.

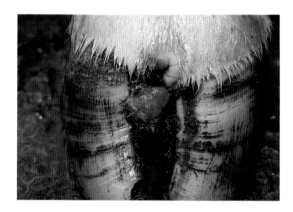

PLATE 5.47 *Proud flesh protruding from a vertical fissure.*

56

HORIZONTAL FISSURE

Horizontal cracks can also occur (Plate 5.48) and often go unnoticed until they have grown down towards the toe. Overeating of concentrates and any severe illness, for example mastitis, metritis or toxaemia, can lead to a total, but temporary, cessation of horn production. When horn formation starts again, movement of hoof continues down over the laminae, but there may be a complete circumferential fissure around the wall of the hoof, relating to the interruption of horn formation.

The cow in Plate 5.48 is a good example of lameness due to horizontal fissures. She had recovered (just!) from an acute *E. coli* mastitis some 5–6 months previously. She was running with the dry cows and starting to put on weight when she developed lameness in all four feet. As the 'thimble' of old horn passed down towards the toe, there was clearly the opportunity for increased movement between the old and new horn and consequently increased opportunity for small stones and other debris to penetrate the crevice and produce infection. Both movement and infection cause pain and lameness, although a significant number

of thimbles simply break off and are shed from the toe, without causing any particular problem. The cow in Plate 5.49 has shed one toe thimble. The other is obviously loose and turned up; this is sometimes referred to as a 'broken toe'.

When lameness occurs, the thimble of loose horn should be removed with a hoof-knife and clippers (not an easy task) and, ideally, a block applied to the sound claw. Sometimes (as in Plate 5.48) all eight claws in all four feet are affected and the cow is probably best culled.

Less severe attacks of laminitis are seen as grooves, circling the front of the hoof as

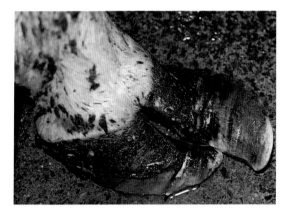

PLATE 5.49   *A horizontal fissure shedding naturally ('broken toe').*

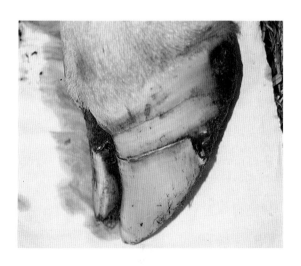

PLATE 5.48   *A horizontal fissure.*

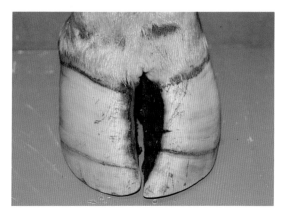

PLATE 5.50   *Hardship lines.*

in Plate 5.50. These have been referred to as hardship lines (27). The date that they were formed (and therefore possibly their cause) can be determined by measuring the distance from the hardship line to the coronary band. Hoof grows at approximately 5mm per month.

FRACTURE OF THE PEDAL BONE

Any severe trauma to the sole of the foot could, in theory, cause a fracture of the pedal bone. The fracture line usually runs from the centre of the pedal joint to the base of the bone (Figure 5.2). Many older cows have a groove running across the articular (joint) surface of the pedal bone, which has been suggested as a predisposing factor to fracture at this site. Oestrus behaviour, with the mounting cow falling heavily onto a rough surface, is one cause. Bones weakened by age, fluorine poisoning or a penetrating infection from the hoof may also fracture.

Typically the medial (inner) claw of the front foot is involved and by adopting a cross-legged stance as in Plate 5.51, weight is transferred onto the sound (lateral) claw. However, the stance alone is not sufficient to indicate a fractured pedal bone. Cows with ulcers in both medial claws will adopt a similar stance.

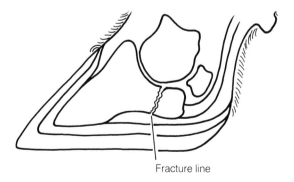

Fracture line

FIGURE 5.2   Fracture of the pedal bone. The fracture line commonly runs from the centre of the pedal joint to the base of the pedal bone.

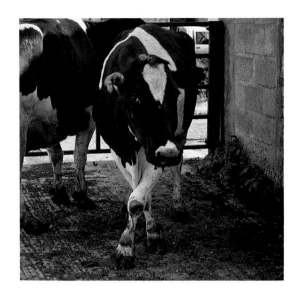

PLATE 5.51   The cross-legged stance of a cow suffering from fracture of the pedal bone.

Affected animals often show little or no heat or swelling of the foot, although there may be pain when the hoof is pinched. Veterinary attention should be sought. The hoof acts as an excellent splint for the pedal bone and provided that a block is applied to the sound claw, many cases heal within 2–3 months.

DRESSINGS, BLOCKS AND SHOES

Hoof Dressing

Opinions vary concerning the value of applying a dressing to a sole ulcer or white line abscess. The disadvantages of a dressing are listed on page 43 and personally I only use a dressing to control haemorrhage after surgery and, in severe cases, in combination with a block. However, resting the affected claw is highly beneficial, promoting healing and improving cow comfort and welfare. The two most commonly used methods are wooden blocks, which are glued to the sole, and nail-on rubber blocks.

Wooden Blocks

Preparation of the hoof, either by thoroughly scraping it with a hoof-knife (Plate 5.52) or by using an electric sander, is the most important part of fixing a wooden block.

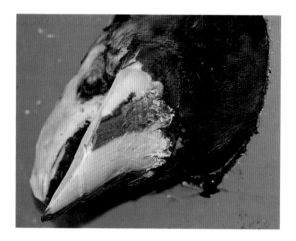

PLATE 5.52   *Clean the hoof before applying the glue for a Demotec wooden block. (64)*

Before the glue is applied, all parts of the hoof should be clean and dry. Even touching the cleaned surfaces with your fingers may produce a greasy surface and reduce adhesion. If the affected claw has a bleeding area it can be difficult to prevent blood splashing onto the claw to be blocked, although attaching a long plastic rectal examination sleeve produces a 'drain' for the blood and helps considerably. Forcing the claws apart with a 5cm length of 7.5mm thick dowelling or a rolled-up wad of paper, improves access to the axial walls and makes gluing easier (Plate 5.53). Mix the glue to a fairly stiff consistency, then apply a layer to the sole, to the sides of the hoof and to the surface of the block to be fixed.

Next push the block firmly onto the sole, and draw the excess glue which is squeezed out, over the sides of the block to improve adhesion. Any remaining glue can be applied to the heel, or if there is

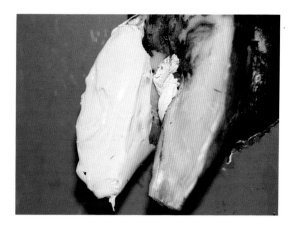

PLATE 5.53   *Apply the glue to the sole and walls. Note the wad of paper forcing the claws apart, thus improving access to the axial wall.*

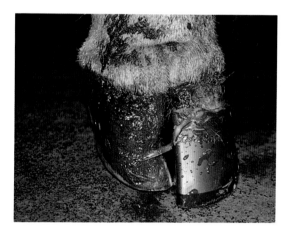

PLATE 5.54   *A glue-on plastic shoe. (Cowslip, Giltspur UK, 63)*

sufficient, to cover the whole block, thereby improving adhesion, strength and weightbearing.

The front tip of the block should be kept at least level with, and perhaps slightly back from, the toe and preferably slightly overlapping the heel, as in Plate 5.55. A block placed too far forward (Figure 5.3) makes the cow walk back on her heels, producing considerable discomfort and uneven and rapid wear of the block.

It is also an advantage not to have the

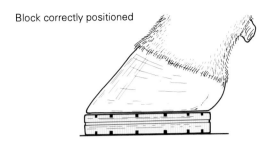
Block correctly positioned

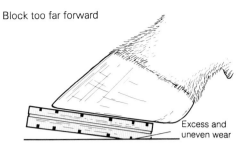
Block too far forward

Excess and
uneven wear

FIGURE 5.3   The wooden block to the right is applied too far forward of the toe. This is uncomfortable, making the cow walk back on her heels.

block overlapping the sole at the sides. Many commercially available blocks seem too large and I regularly cut off a sliver (Figure 5.4) to make them smaller. This uses less glue and improves adhesion.

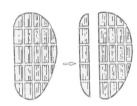
FIGURE 5.4   Many commercial blocks are too wide, and removal of a sliver improves adhesion.

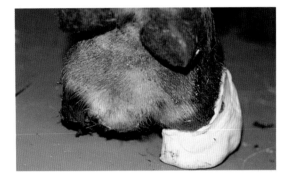
PLATE 5.55   *The glue fully covers the block. The affected claw is well off the ground.*

PVC Shoes

PVC shoes (Cowslips, Giltspur Ltd, see Plate 5.54 and ref. 63) are applied following similar cleaning of the foot. They have advantages over wooden blocks in that the glue is mixed in the shoe, the PVC heel is slower to wear away than a wooden block and the side wall of the shoe supports the hoof. Most importantly, the glue sets quickly, even in cold weather. As with wooden blocks, it is essential that the PVC shoe is pushed far enough back to support the heel. With Cowslips this may entail some trimming of the sound claw prior to application. If correctly applied, both PVC shoes and wooden blocks should stay on for at least two months, during which time it is remarkable how quite severe lesions will heal. However, if the heel is becoming worn, then the PVC

shoe or block should be removed, because walking will be uncomfortable.

Rubber Blocks

Rubber blocks are nailed on (Plate 5.56). They are cheaper and easier to apply, but not universally popular because of the danger of nails penetrating through the white line, leading to infection. Moreover, they do not stay on as long as glued blocks and when they fall off, there is a risk of solar penetration by the shed nails.

Figure 5.5 shows the importance of the positioning of the nails. 'A' will pass through the white line and with its bevelled edge deflecting it outwards will pass out through the wall, totally avoiding all sensitive tissues. However, 'B' is well inside the white line and

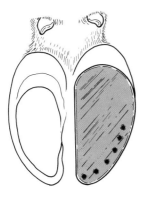
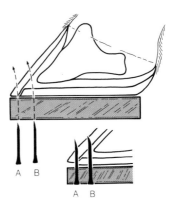

FIGURE 5.5   The correct positioning of nails for a rubber block. A nail inserted into the white line at 'A' will pass out through the hoof wall without damaging sensitive tissues. 'B' is passing inside the white line and will penetrate the corium, leading to infection, pain and lameness.

although it will still reappear on the side of the wall to be clinched over, it has penetrated the corium en route and this will lead to infection, pain and lameness.

Before applying the block, ensure that the sole has been trimmed to provide a sound and level weightbearing surface and that there are no lesions present which could in themselves produce lameness. Hold the foot firmly and hammer the nails, bevelled edge innermost, through the white line area of the sole. With its one-sided bevel, the mail will curve outwards slightly, to reappear through the wall where it can be clinched over. Lubrication of the mails assists their penetration. It is often easiest to insert the first nail towards the toe, to establish the

position of the block and the second towards the heel. The remaining nail holes should then be in the correct position.

Plastic Protective Shoes

Plastic protective shoes (Plate 5.57) were once popular. They were secured by tying them tightly at the fetlock, encasing both hooves. A dressing could be applied to the affected claw. Shoes were available with a block on the left or right side, thus lifting the affected claw and reducing its weightbearing. However, they are less popular now, partly because they are difficult to secure and partly because the foot tends to become damp and sweaty inside the shoe, thus retarding healing.

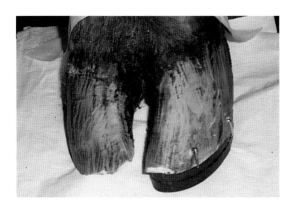

PLATE 5.56   A rubber nail-on block.

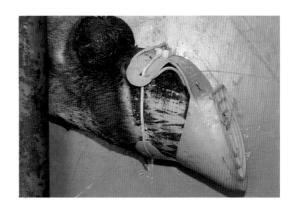

PLATE 5.57   A plastic protective shoe.

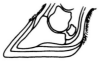

CHAPTER SIX

The Causes and Prevention of Lameness

In a herd with a lameness problem, it is unlikely that there will be a single cause involved. Lameness is a true example of a multifactorial condition, that is, there will be a number of factors producing an adverse effect on hoof condition. Each factor on its own may not produce lameness. However, when acting in concert, severe foot problems can result.

Some of the adverse influences on lameness would be very difficult to avoid. Typical examples include calving, which has been shown to produce solar haemorrhages (27) and weaken the white line (40); standing on hard concrete surfaces (20); and the high level of feeding required for commercial milk production (21). However, the effects can be minimised by ensuring that those factors which we are able to influence are optimal for cattle hoof care.

Although the influence of nutritional, environmental, management and toxic factors on lameness will be considered separately, it is important that the reader appreciates that in reality all these will be acting in concert. The major importance of calving as a factor rendering the corium more fragile and therefore more susceptible to nutritional and environmental factors cannot be overstressed. This is discussed on page 75.

In this chapter the word laminitis is loosely used to include changes in the sole (where there are papillae and no laminae) and in the white line (which has neither laminae nor papillae and primarily consists of intertubular horn). Generalised changes in the corium (coriitis or coriosis) (38) might be a better term (see page 14). Detailed scientific reviews of the causes of sole lesions in cattle are available elsewhere (15, 46, 56).

NUTRITIONAL FACTORS

Acidosis

It is generally accepted that high starch:low fibre diets, producing ruminal acidosis, are the most important nutritional factors in the production of laminitis and this can result in lameness due to sole ulcers and white line abscesses. Rations should be formulated with a concentrate:forage ratio no greater than 60:40. Even at this level problems can occur, especially if the concentrate is high in starch and the silage is precision chopped, high in quality and low in fibre, giving an overall neutral detergent fibre level in the ration of less than 40%. Such diets benefit from the inclusion of 1–2kg of straw, either mixed, as in a complete ration, or simply made available on free access. It is surprising how much straw cows will eat if it is available on free access, and dry fibrous foods seem to stimulate better salivation and rumination than moist forages such as silage. The long fibre of big bale silage is a useful alternative. The normal rumen pH is around 6.5. After a feed of concentrate in the parlour this may fall to 6.0 or even 5.5 if a large intake of a high starch (i.e. high energy) concentrate is received. Starch is fermented by the ruminal micro-organisms into lactic acid and the fall in rumen pH is known as rumen acidosis. While substantial quantities of lactic acid can be converted into propionate and then into glucose, if overloading occurs, lactic acid leaks into adjacent blood vessels. Initially it is buffered by bicarbonate, but increasing amounts of lactic acid produce a metabolic acidosis. This means that the blood itself starts to become too acid and affected cows may pant, trying to breathe off the excess acid.

In herds with acidosis there may be an increased incidence of regurgitation of the cud and of tail-swishing due to vaginal irritation from acid urine.

Bacterial Endotoxins

The precise way in which acidosis causes laminitis is still unknown. It has been suggested that the change in rumen fermentation causes the release of bacterial endotoxins (endotoxins are breakdown products of dead bacteria) which, when absorbed, stimulate histamine release by the cow (2). Histamine damages blood vessels, thus disturbing the delicate blood flow control mechanisms within the hoof, described on page 10. Pooling of blood occurs and blood clots (thrombosis) may form.

It is probable that damage to the arteriovenous anastomoses, the minute connections between arteries and veins which exist at the base of the laminae and papillae, is involved in the basic changes of laminitis (59). If there is insufficient blood flow in the corium, this leads to inadequate supplies of oxygen and sulphur-containing amino acids, both of which are essential for horn formation. It has been shown experimentally that changes occur in the corium as soon as two hours after injecting lactic acid into the rumen (29). Within seven days there were microscopic areas of separation between the horn and the horn-forming layers (viz. between the stratum corneum and stratum germinativum) (see page 5). If allowed to progress, this could lead to sole ulcers or even total horizontal fissures as described on page

Bacterial endotoxins are not only formed in the rumen. They can also arise from bacterial death following acute mastitis or metritis (uterine infection) and both conditions therefore require adequate treatment in order to prevent subsequent hoof disorders. Changes in the blood circulation around the time of calving often lead to a pooling of fluid. This is commonly seen in the udder as excess oedema or 'nature'. A similar pooling of fluid occurs in the corium, leading to softer horn production and, in more extreme cases, to haemorrhage, horn separation and sole ulcers. The problem is exacerbated by the fact that heifers especially have been shown to spend longer periods standing during the two weeks prior to and the two weeks following calving (37). Disease at this stage, leading to yet further pooling of fluid in the corium, is therefore particularly important. Cubicle comfort is also important and this is referred to on pages 68-71.

The maintenance of good blood flow within the foot is assisted by exercise. Make sure that cows at calving are not totally confined to calving boxes and, if sick, encourage them to move around a little. This does not, of course, mean putting them back into the main herd where they would have to compete for food and priority in the pecking order.

Rumen acidosis is, to a certain extent, a self-perpetuating process. Decreasing rumen pH decreases rumen motility, which in turn depresses appetite and consequently dry matter intake falls. The cow that has over-eaten concentrate in the parlour will therefore probably eat less forage, thus exacerbating rumen acidosis. This is particularly important immediately after calving, when the cow's appetite is depressed generally and reduction in forage intake is often exacerbated by increased concentrate intakes. The substitution rate (decrease in kg silage DM eaten per 1kg extra concentrate given) is much greater in early lactation, and hence increased concentrate intakes depress forage consumption.

Frequency of Feeding

On twice daily milking, parlour concentrate intakes should be restricted to 8 – 10kg per day, i.e. a maximum of 5kg per feed, and ideally 4kg per feed, or less. There is a high risk of laminitis at parlour intakes of 12kg per day and above, especially if a high starch product is used.

The practice of dispensing out-of-parlour feeds of concentrate (or maize gluten, palm kernel, etc.) during morning milking should also be discouraged. Distributing the feed when the cows are shut in for milking may be easier, but it means that the cows will then be faced with a second feed of concentrates as soon as they leave the parlour. Some of

the high yielders may not eat any of the out-of-parlour concentrate and hence yields suffer, while the stale milkers get overfat. Those fresh calvers which do eat the concentrate run the risk of an even more severe acidosis and hence feet and fertility may both be affected. Concentrates containing increased levels of digestible fibre will help.

However, it is far better to feed concentrates equally throughout the day, either as a complete diet through a forage waggon, or as 1 – 2 additional feeds outside the parlour.

Dietary Fat

Avoid high fat rations. Levels of fat in excess of 4% of the total dry matter can lead to depressed forage digestion due to the ruminal micro-organisms becoming coated with fat. This could produce a secondary acidosis.

Changes in Diet at Calving

Sudden changes in diet are also dangerous, especially if from low to high concentrate rations. This may occur at calving. Ideally, cows should be fed a small quantity (to avoid them becoming too fat) of the production ration prior to calving, to acclimatise the rumen micro-organisms and then, following calving, the ration should be built up slowly, so that peak concentrate intakes are not reached until 2 – 3 weeks into lactation. Flat-rate feeding, whereby cows are fed a maximum level of concentrate (usually 8 – 9kg per day), irrespective of level of yield, has probably helped to reduce foot problems in some herds, by restricting peak concentrate intakes. However, in other herds where all the concentrate is fed **outside** the parlour and cows are introduced immediately onto maximum ration following an all-forage restricted diet in the dry period, flat-rate feeding may be counter-productive and this might explain why some people (60) have found an increased incidence of lameness in flat-rate feeding herds. This is a good example of the multifactorial influences on lameness, discussed in the introduction to this chapter.

It is the composition of the diet and not simply the overall energy intake which affects the incidence of laminitis. Table 6.1 (39) shows two groups of cows, one of which (A) was fed a high fibre diet and the other (B) a low fibre and high concentrate diet. Both rations had the same overall crude protein (CP) content and both groups of cows achieved a similar total daily energy intake (MJ/kg), although the high fibre group clearly needed a greater dry matter intake to do so.

The high incidence of both laminitis and sole ulcers in the low fibre group (B) is most striking. Despite regular foot-trimming, group B also had a higher incidence of solar overgrowths. In this trial, precalving feeding had no effect.

Similar results (Table 6.2) have been reported (49) in a trial which continued over two lactations, the differences in the concentrate and forage diets being greater in the second lactation, presumably because of an additive effect of first lactation insults.

High concentrate feeding is not the only factor involved in the production of white line abscess and sole ulcers however, as there has been a high incidence of both conditions in a herd fed a low level of concentrate on a flat-rate system, giving an overall concentrate:forage ratio of only 20:80 (6).

TABLE 6.1 Two groups of cows* having the same total daily protein energy intake, but Group A was fed a high fibre diet and Group B a low fibre diet (39).

	ME (MJ/kg)	CP (g/kg)	No. showing clinical laminitis	No. showing sole ulcers
Group A fed a high fibre diet	10.8	158	2 (8%)	2 (8%)
Group B fed a low fibre diet	11.1	157	17 (68%)	16 (64%)

* Number of cows in Group A = 26 and in Group B = 25

TABLE 6.2 The number of cows treated for sole ulcers on high concentrate and high fibre diets. In Experiment 1 concentrates and forage (roughage) were fed separately and at the end of the first lactation high concentrate fed cows were switched onto a high forage diet and vice versa. In Experiment 2 concentrates and forage were fed as a complete diet to all cows and there was no change at the end of the first lactation (49).

	1st lactation No. of cows	1st lactation No. treated	2nd lactation No. of cows	2nd lactation No. treated
		%		%
Experiment 1				
High concentrate group	46	26 (58)	29	19 (66)
High roughage group	47	14 (30)	35	11 (31)
		0.005 <P<0.01		0.005 <P<0.01
Experiment 2				
High concentrate group	33	8 (24)	14	12 (85)
High roughage group	30	5 (17)	20	6 (28)
		NS		P<0.005

Significance between groups statistically tested by Pearson's x^2 test using the hypothesis that yes or no sole ulcer is equally distributed among both groups
NS Not significant

Dietary Protein

Diets high in protein have been suggested as possibly causing an increased incidence of lameness (5, 42) perhaps due to high levels of ammonia produced in the rumen (60), but this is not thought to be a common problem. The very high protein intakes in association with spring grazing certainly do not seem to be a major cause. It is possible that high protein winter rations are associated with high concentrate intakes and it is in fact starch overload and not excess protein which is the factor involved. Diets giving an overall crude protein of above 18% should be avoided however.

High incidences of lameness are often associated with grass silage, especially if the silage is wet and poorly fermented. Whether this is due to toxic substances (possibly amines) in the silage having a direct effect on laminitis, or whether it is simply due to the fact that feeding such silage reduces overall forage intake, thus altering the concentrate:forage ratio, is not known (27).

Feeding During Rearing

In heifers, high levels of concentrates, and especially a sudden change from low to high concentrate even during the rearing period (i.e. less than 18 months old), have been shown to produce laminitis (27).

Feed intakes to produce growth rates of 800g per day and above were found to produce sole haemorrhages in heifers. This is particularly interesting, considering that over the past 10–15 years there has been a marked change towards calving dairy heifers at two years old and, to achieve this, increased growth rates which require higher concentrate feeding, have been necessary. Could this be one reason why there has been an increase in lameness over the same period?

Some herds have recently reduced concentrate intakes for heifer rearing in an attempt to alleviate this. Provided that forage is made freely available, growth rates do not appear to suffer. Ration palatability, and hence overall dry matter intakes, can be maximised by incorporating brewers grains and similar high digestibility fibre feeds. Post-calving dry matter intakes may be higher in heifers which have been reared on high forage diets.

Cow Condition

Cow condition at calving is also important. Cows overfat at calving have reduced appetites, particularly for forage (26), and are therefore more prone to developing acidosis and laminitis. Ideally, cows should be fed to be **dried off** at condition score 2.5–3.0 and maintained in this condition until calving.

If overfat at drying off, it is extremely difficult to produce significant weight loss during the dry period. A diet of ad lib barley straw plus 0.5kg fishmeal will lead to weight loss, but of course it is highly inefficient in terms of feed utilisation to allow cows to gain excess weight and then force them to lose it again. Silage should never be fed ad lib to dry cows unless weight gain is specifically required.

Zinc, Sulphur and Biotin

Specific nutrients have been suggested to increase the hardness of hoof horn, but documented evidence of their effectiveness is often contradictory and their importance compared with other factors is likely to be limited.

Soft horn is said to have a higher water content and lower zinc and sulphur content than hard horn. Supplementation with 3g per day zinc oxide has been suggested as being beneficial, although zinc methionine may be better absorbed and more efficiently incorporated into the hoof. There is a risk that oversupplementation with zinc or sulphur will induce copper deficiency.

The addition of biotin to the ration has also been suggested to decrease lameness and improve the rate of healing of sole ulcers. Biotin is certainly considered to improve hoof condition in both horses and pigs, but sufficient biotin should be produced by the ruminal micro-organisms for the cow's needs. However, a Japanese study found a relationship between blood biotin levels and cattle lameness and recommended dietary supplementation with biotin (34).

Once the corium has suffered one attack of laminitis, it never fully recovers. Miroscopic changes including fibrosis, occlusion of blood vessels and other factors which reduce the functional capacity of the corium often persist (41). This is probably one reason why, when the cows have been through a laminitic insult, they have bad feet for the remainder of their lives. The hooves may remain chronically misshapen (Plate 2.11 is a good example) and have to be regularly trimmed in an attempt to restore reasonable shape and weightbearing surfaces. Long-term changes to the pedal bone may also occur (58), including irregular projections (exostoses) from its lower surface, which may lead to discomfort when walking. A typical example is shown in Plate 5.25.

ENVIRONMENTAL FACTORS

Lying Times

Environment has a major impact on lameness, in that cows which spend long periods standing are often the worst affected. Long periods standing produce increased pressure on the sole, thereby leading to physical traumatic damage, often manifest as haemorrhage in the typical sole ulcer site. In addition, if a cow stands but does not move, the delicate blood flow mechanisms within the foot (see page 10) are put under stress, the blood pools and stagnates and horn formation is affected.

Ideally, a cow should spend between 12 and 14 hours per day lying down (16, 31, 33) and to achieve this, cubicles must be well designed and well bedded.

Table 6.3 shows the amount of time that cows spent lying down each day in cubicles which were of identical design but differently bedded. Another trial (20) comparing two identically managed herds, both housed in identical cubicles, showed that using more straw bedding in the cubicles increased the amount of

lying time, that more first-lactation heifers* went into the cubicle house and that the time between entry and lying down was shortened. This led to a significant decrease in the incidence of sole ulcers and white line infection in the herd where ample straw bedding was in use.

Whatever the cubicle design therefore, adequate bedding, whether it be mats, sawdust or deep straw, is essential for comfort. Mats should ideally be covered with sawdust or straw to keep them dry and hence reduce the risk of sores developing on legs (and to reduce the risk of mastitis). Second-hand quarry belting, fixed with its worn surface downwards, makes reasonable quality and inexpensive cubicle matting. Deep straw is obviously ideal, but it can sometimes be difficult to get clean straw to adhere to a concrete cubicle base. This can be overcome by putting 4 to 6 inches of rotting straw yard muck into the cubicle base and covering it with clean straw. The cows soon compress the muck down to 1 to 1.5 inches thick and at the same time it dries and sticks to the cubicle base, thereby acting as a 'key' for further straw bedding. This system also provides excellent padding for the cow's knees, when she is putting maximum weight on them as she rises to stand (see Figure 6.2).

Outbreaks of lameness are often seen when cows which have been housed in straw yards are transferred into cubicles. The cows find the cubicles strange and less comfortable, lying times decrease, trauma to the hoof is increased and lameness results.

One of the worst outbreaks of lameness (sole ulcer and white line disease) I have experienced was associated with just such a situation. The straw-housed cows were transferred into a new cubicle house, the floors of which had been laid so that the front half was flat and the rear had a

TABLE 6.3 In this trial it was found that cows preferred cubicles which were either deeply bedded with chopped straw or had a thick cushioned mat (7).

Type of cubicle bed	Length of time cows spent resting each day
Bare concrete	7.2 hours
Insulated concrete screed	8.1 hours
Hard rubber mat	9.8 hours
Chopped straw on concrete	14.1 hours
Proprietary cow cushion	14.4 hours

* Heifers are more likely to be bullied by cows and therefore less likely to enter a cubicle house if there is no escape route. They are also more prone to sole ulcers and hence this is the reason why the researchers specifically targeted this group.

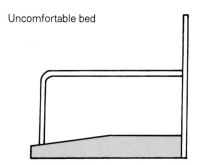 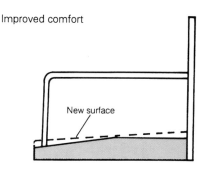

FIGURE 6.1   Cubicles with a change in slope in the centre of the bed are much less comfortable.

steep slope, producing a ridge in the centre of the lying area (Figure 6.1). The cubicles were obviously uncomfortable and very few cows used them properly. Many were standing, while others were lying half in the cubicle and half in the dunging passage, or totally lying in the dunging passage. When the beds were relaid, with an even 4 inch fall from front to rear, cubicle usage increased and eventually the lameness subsided. Those cows which had severe ulcers never fully recovered and many had to be culled.

Cubicle Design

Overall cubicle size and the design of the divisions all have an effect on cow comfort. Cubicles should be at least 1.21 m wide and 2.2 m long (approximately 4 ft × 7 ft) (32) and, if possible, allowing another 1–1.2 m at the front for a lunging space, that is an area into which a cow can move her head when getting up. Figure 6.2 shows the movements a cow makes when standing and the need for the forward space.

Length is probably the most important dimension and seems to have the greatest effect on cow acceptance.

The cubicle should provide sufficient forward space for the cow to extend her neck when regurgitating the cud (33). If a cow is forced to sit with her head to one side and with pressure on her rumen from the side divisions of an undersized cubicle, she may need to stand, front feet in the cubicle and hind feet in the dunging passage, in order to ruminate properly. Excessive standing and corrosive slurry can both lead to foot problems.

Avoid excessively high cubicle steps, because cows do not like reversing out of a cubicle and stepping down. Steps 6 inches high or greater could lead to cubicle rejection.

Width requirements are to a certain extent affected by cubicle design, in that narrow cubicles can be partly offset by divisions which allow space sharing.

I prefer to see the minimum of cubicle division, and the Dutch Comfort type shown in Figure 6.3 is good for comfort. The standard Newton Rigg cubicle (Figure 6.4) perhaps has the disadvantage of two vertical bars at the rear which can

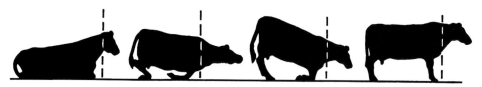

FIGURE 6.2   A cow may lunge forwards for a distance of 1–2m when rising naturally.

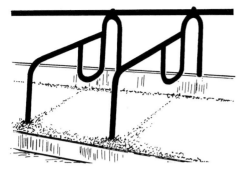

FIGURE 6.3   Cubicles such as Dutch Comfort (above) or cantilever types with a minimum of division between them are often more comfortable.

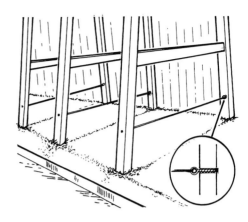

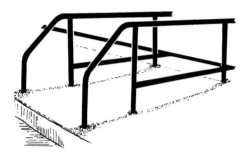

FIGURE 6.4   Newton Rigg cubicles bedded with straw.

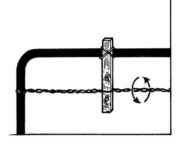

FIGURE 6.6   The lower cubicle rail can be replaced by a rope under tension. In the lower diagram a two-stranded rope is brought under tension by rotating a piece of wood (see arrows) fixed between the two strands. When the rope is taut, the wood is tied to the top cubicle rail.

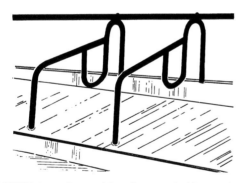

FIGURE 6.5   Second-hand quarry belting makes a good cubicle mat, thus increasing cow comfort and lying times.

cause damage to the cow's pelvis. The Newton Rigg cubicles were well-bedded, but additional cow comfort and increased lying times were obtained by using a strip of second-hand quarry belting as a cow

mat (Figure 6.5). The matting must be continued to the rear lip of the cubicle of course, to prevent hock damage. A length of rope under tension can be used in place of the lower cubicle rail (Figure 6.6). The square edges of the wooden uprights in these cubicles could lead to injury.

Standard heights quoted (1) are 400 mm for the lower rail and 1,050 mm for the top rail. In Plate 6.1 the cubicle beds had been recently concreted, thus decreasing the distance between floor and rail, and cows damaged their hocks, leading to hock swellings (Plate 6.2), abscesses, general discomfort and a further reluctance to use the cubicles. If cubicle divisions are insufficient however, cows

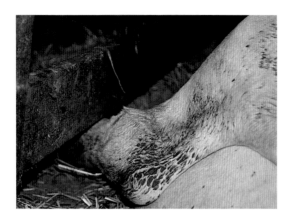

PLATE 6.1   The lower cubicle rail is too low and will damage the cows' hocks.

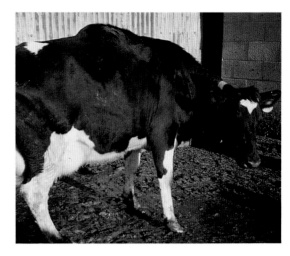

PLATE 6.3   Haematoma on a cow's back caused by poor cubicle design.

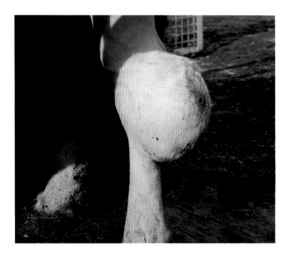

PLATE 6.2   Hock swelling and abscess.

may try to pass underneath and get trapped. This is what happened to the cow in Plate 6.3, who subsequently developed a haematoma (blood blister) on her back.

The position of the front neck rail is critical. Too far forward and the cow can still dung on the cubicle bed when she stands up, thereby increasing the risk of mastitis. Too far back or too low and the rail makes the cubicle so uncomfortable that cows start to lie in the passageways, thus exacerbating lameness.

Although most neck rails are fixed to the top of the cubicle division, this is not the ideal siting. A rail, positioned 4 – 6 inches lower than the withers of a standing cow, as in Figure 6.7, will increase cubicle acceptance without producing excessive soiling of the beds. Brisket boards are also useful if positioned correctly.

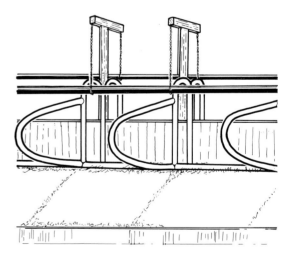

FIGURE 6.7   A heavy metal rail suspended 4 – 6 inches lower than the withers height of a standing cow is better than a conventional neck rail which is often fixed to the top of the cubicle division.

70

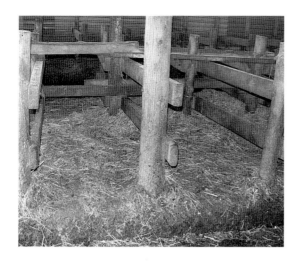

FIGURE 6.8 Excessively narrow home-made cubicles. The cows found these uncomfortable.

Heifer Training

Training heifers to use cubicles is important. After the stress of calving, they have enough to cope with — learning a new system of feeding, entering the milking parlour and establishing their position in the pecking order — without finding that there is nowhere comfortable to lie down! If heifers cannot be reared in cubicles, house them for 4–6 weeks in the summer, whilst the cows are still at grazing. An alternative is to mix heifers with the main herd, or even just the dry cows, for 3–4 weeks before calving. It is a nuisance if non-lactating heifers enter a herring-bone milking parlour, of course, but having to deal with lame heifers on a regular basis is likely to be equally as time-consuming.

Cow Behaviour

In addition to cubicle comfort, there must be enough space for cows to move around. Overcrowding and inadequate loafing areas could mean insufficient exercise and consequently poor blood flow within the feet, especially during cold weather. A similar syndrome (known as 'trench foot') affected soldiers standing for long periods in muddy trenches during the First World War.

Some of the narrowest cubicles I have ever seen were home-made, using heavy timbers, and fitted into an existing building. The cubicles were of varying sizes, with some as narrow as 910mm (3ft) wide (Figure 6.8). The head of a bolt used to attach the lower rail protruded into the restricted space and was worn smooth from the cows continually knocking against it. The owner admitted that the cows did not like using these cubicles!

Existing cubicle houses can be successfully modified by constructing new cubicles in a herring-bone arrangement. This allows both increased width and length without the need to make any changes to the curb and passageway.

In one trial (47) where preference for cubicle design was assessed by recording the length of time that each cubicle was used, Dutch Comfort and improved Dutch Comfort cubicles were found to be superior to basic Newton Rigg. The different designs are shown in Figure 6.9. However, in this trial, once a cow had accepted a particular cubicle type, the length of time spent lying was the same, irrespective of cubicle design.

For low-ranking cows, cubicles can act as both a lying area and a safey zone, in that the side bars increase their effective personal space (50). There is general agreement that there should be sufficient cubicles to allow all cows to lie down at the same time, i.e. at least equal numbers of cows and cubicles (57).

Systems should also be designed with 'escape routes'. If cubicle passages are blind-ended, heifers will be reluctant to enter because of the fear of being trapped by older cows, and hence lying times may decrease. Ideally there should be escape routes approximately every 12 cubicles. A narrow gap, just wide enough to allow a heifer to pass from one cubicle passageway to the next, is sufficient.

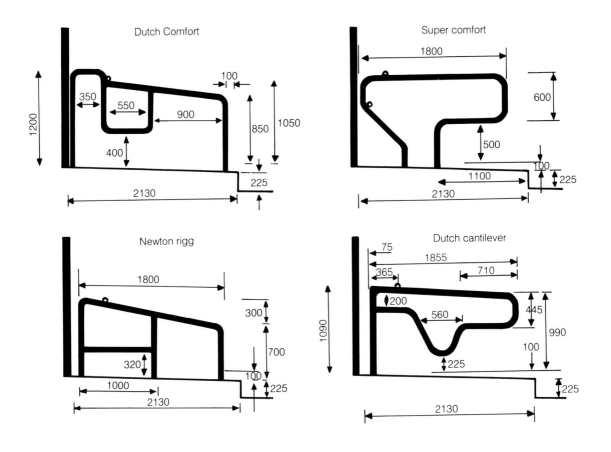

FIGURE 6.9   A range of cubicle designs with measurements given in mm. *(Dr. J. O'Connell, Moorepark)*

Decreased lying times are particularly critical immediately after calving. Heifers retained in a separate group for their first lactation give much better yields than their counterparts introduced directly into the main herd (23). Foot health could be contributing to these improved yields.

Avoid sharp turns. An animal normally turns a corner by walking slowly around it. If corners are sharp, or if heifers (especially) have to make sudden avoiding flight movements to escape from aggressor cows, turning will probably be achieved by pivoting on the sole of the foot. This has the effect of forcing the wall away from the sole, thus expanding the width of the white line and weakening it.

A large number of cows jostling for position behind out-of-parlour feeders can have a similar effect. Feeders are best spaced well away from each other, to reduce competition.

Keep the areas beside feed troughs clean and free from waste silage. Cows continually standing on waste silage may not wear their front feet sufficiently, and claw overgrowth may result.

MANAGEMENT FACTORS

Although the design of housing systems is important, the way in which cows are managed in those systems can also influence lameness.

Wet Conditions and Slurry

Wet conditions underfoot can lead to rapid softening of the hoof. This is common knowledge to us all: the best time to cut your toenails is just after you have had a bath! Overcrowded conditions will reduce lying times (62), especially if cubicles are small and uncomfortable. Normal horn should contain about 15% moisture, but this can almost double if the feet are continually in wet conditions. This weakens the hooves considerably (but makes them easier to trim!).

Accumulated stale and corrosive slurry can increase the incidence of heel necrosis or digital dermatitis (9), especially if cows are tightly housed with a high stocking density. Cubicle passages should be scraped twice daily and stale areas of slurry avoided. The once or twice weekly sprinkling of slaked lime, used in cubicles for mastitis prevention, is probably also beneficial, in that it can harden and dry the hooves (12).

Rough Surfaces

Damaged and pitted concrete can cause excessive bruising to the sole and can give rise to small stones which can become impacted in the white line. Such concrete should therefore be repaired. When concrete is laid, a small round aggregate should be used and the mix kept dry. Wet mixes tend to wear more easily at the surface, thus exposing the aggregate. Flint aggregates should not be used. Their sharp edges are even more likely to traumatise the sole.

Cows which have to walk long distances along flint gravel tracks will be particularly prone to white line disease and sole penetration. Both conditions have been shown to be more common in the summer (53, 55). If given the option, cows will use specific tracks when walking in and out to pasture. We have all seen the foot marks and areas commonly favoured; often these are at the edge of the much harder tractor route (Plate 6.4),

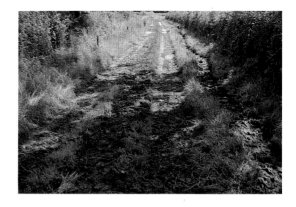

PLATE 6.4 *Favoured tracks at the side of a roadway. Cows prefer walking on a soft surface.*

which is in the centre of the roadway.

It has also been shown (17) that cows which are rushed along tracks, e.g. by pushing them with a tractor or using a dog, do not use or produce 'cow favoured areas' and in these herds lameness is increased. Gentle handling so that the cow can avoid unsuitable surfaces and place her feet in her preferred position is therefore important. Lame cows usually congregate at the rear of the herd. If the cows are being pushed ahead by an impatient stockman, it is these cows especially which become tightly packed and are unable to use favoured tracks. Such behaviour obviously also has important welfare implications.

Cow Tracks

Specific walking surfaces for cows have been constructed alongside the concrete or stone roadways used for tractors. Examples are shown in Figure 6.10 and Plate 6.5. A trench 1 metre wide and 0.3 metre deep is lined with a type of geotextile membrane used in road construction. A drainage pipe is run along the base and the trench is then filled with stone aggregate, preferably with finer stone towards the surface. This is then covered with a second, reinforced geotextile membrane, with the edges of

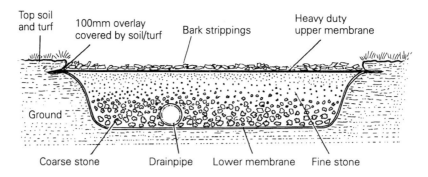

Top soil and turf 100mm overlay covered by soil/turf Bark strippings Heavy duty upper membrane

Ground

Coarse stone Drainpipe Lower membrane Fine stone

Dimensions: 1m wide, 300mm deep, 200mm coarse stones, 50–100mm bark strippings or cundy peelings

FIGURE 6.10   Cow tracks need to be both well drained and comfortable. They improve cow comfort, increase speed of walking and reduce lameness. (*John Hughes*)

the membranes being covered by soil to hold them in position. Finally a 50 to 100 mm layer of bark chippings or cundy wood peelings is placed on the surface.

Being well drained, the track always stays clean and in good condition. Although only 1 metre wide and thus allowing only single file walking, the track is so comfortable that cows move quite quickly and overall cow transit times are often less than if they were walking three to four abreast along a rough stone roadway. The reduction in trauma to the sole is bound to be beneficial, especially in the freshly calved animal.

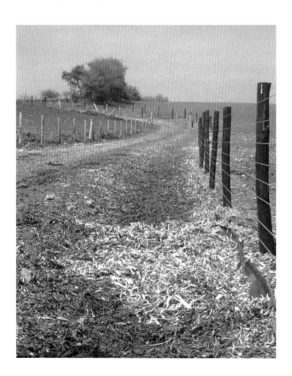

PLATE 6.5   A specially made cow track.

Excessive Exercise

Whilst excessive standing reduces blood flow in the hoof and is detrimental, excessive walking can lead to overwearing of the soles, which become soft and easily bruised. This soft sole syndrome is a common cause of lameness in heifers and also in young bulls introduced into a cubicle-housed dairy herd. A heavy workload, resulting in excess wear on the hind feet, plus a reluctance to use cubicles (because of their size) often leads to lameness in bulls.

On lifting the foot, the sole is found to be worn so soft that it can be easily depressed with the thumb. Sometimes a white line infection is also present, especially at the toe. Bulls used in cubicle housed dairy herds should therefore be rested in a straw yard or loosebox, ideally for at least one week in three.

If, on examination of the foot of first calved heifers, the sole can be depressed by thumb pressure, they should similarly be housed in a straw yard for 2–4 weeks. Failure to do this could result in the development of sole ulcers and sole penetration, in addition to the obvious welfare implications.

However, it is also possible to underwear hooves. The hooves of heifers reared and housed continuously on straw or in sand yards simply do not get adequate wear. This leads to overgrowth at the toe, a backward rotation of the hoof and pedal bone, pain, discomfort and a predisposition to sole ulcers, as described on pages 10 to 12.

Such animals should be given a strip of clean concrete against the feed face, sufficient in width to accommodate all four feet when standing eating. This will then allow normal wear of the hooves. If overgrown front feet are seen, a sprinkling of sand on the concrete produces even better wear. Similar considerations apply to milking cows, of course.

If waste silage is continually present when they are standing at the feed face, this could lead to overgrown front feet. Keeping the area clean and applying a sprinkling of sand once a week could help keep the hooves in better shape. I think this would appeal to all of us who have had to trim front feet.

Dry Cows

Cows should be taken off concrete and, ideally, put out onto pasture during the dry period (44). Movement through grass helps to keep the hooves clean and heel horn has an opportunity to regrow, thus alleviating the effects of heel necrosis and slurry heel. The cow also has ample opportunity to lie down. She has a comfortable bed and during the dry period does not need to spend long periods standing and eating. Not only does this improve foot condition, but it also gives an opportunity for the traumatic injuries to knees, hocks and pelvis, shown in Plates 6.2 and 6.6, to recover.

If winter conditions do not allow dry cows to be left at pasture, then at least house them in straw yards. If cubicles are inherently uncomfortable, they will be even worse for large, heavily-pregnant cows.

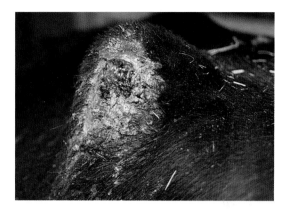

PLATE 6.6 Discharge from a fractured wing of the pelvis originally caused by cubicle damage.

TOXIC AND MISCELLANEOUS FACTORS

Any acute toxic illness can lead to horn production being slowed down or even stopped temporarily, depending on the severity of the illness. In previous chapters it has been shown that this produces changes in the hoof wall varying from hardship lines (Plate 5.50) to a complete horizontal fissure (Plate 5.48). Examples of illnesses include peracute mastitis, acute toxic metritis, photosensitisation and foot and mouth disease.

Changes at Calving

Many people have described an association between calving and the production of sole haemorrhage and other causes of laminitis (27, 40, 46), and lameness generally is more common during the first few months after calving (*54*). The precise cause of this is unknown, but the rings on a cow's horns indicate that there is a disruption in horn formation in every cow at calving.

This is clearly shown in the cow in Plate 6.7. Although 13 years old, she had had only six calves and hence the six rings on her horns. If you look at a bull's horns you will not find any rings (unless he has been very sick at some stage). This disruption in horn formation also occurs in the foot and it means that at the time of calving the corium is very fragile and even more susceptible to bruising. Yet this is often the time when many other stresses are imposed on the cow, for example a sudden change to an 'acidosis type' ration, or an introduction into a new (and perhaps uncomfortable) cubicle house, both of which are in themselves important causes of foot problems.

A small but increasing number of dairy farmers are attempting to minimise stress by keeping heifers in straw yards for the first 4 to 6 weeks after calving. Most agree that this leads to:

- decreased lameness, because lying times are increased and so there is less trauma on an inherently fragile corium
- increased yields, presumably because the heifers are more comfortable
- improved cubicle acceptance when the heifers are eventually introduced into cubicles. This is perhaps the most surprising aspect of the system, but probably emphasises the fact that calving is a much more stressful procedure than we imagine

The cause of the disruption of horn formation at calving is unknown. The blood levels of haptoglobulins and other acute phase proteins (which are indicators of inflammation) increase at parturition, and the signal for parturition to start is in fact the intra-uterine release of cortisone by the calf. As administration of cortisone to horses can induce laminitis, perhaps it is the foetal cortisone that is important.

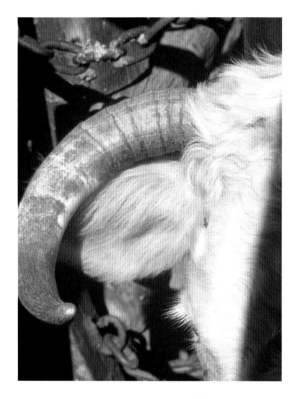

PLATE 6.7 *The rings on a cow's horns are due to disruption of horn formation at the time of calving. Similar changes occur within the feet.*

Another theory is that it is the start of lactation rather than the process of calving which is involved. Sulphur-containing amino acids are needed for both keratin formation (see page 5) and for milk production. The sudden start of milk production, draining all the sulphur amino acids away from horn formation and into lactation, could result in a short period of poor quality horn formation. There is also a drop in serum protein levels around the time of calving. This leads to oedema (the accumulation of fluid) under the skin of the udder and belly: perhaps similar changes could occur within the foot, with stasis of blood leading to anoxia and poor horn formation, as described on page 15.

76

Mastitis and the other toxic changes mentioned above are also more common immediately after calving.

Changes in management and feeding are in themselves of primary importance. For example, in one experiment, 10 steers were housed, fed and managed with a group of 10 pregnant heifers of the same age. As the heifers calved, changed housing and were transferred onto a production ration the steers followed suit (obviously only the heifers calved!). Both steers and heifers in the group showed sole haemorrhages, although the haemorrhages were more severe in the heifers. This shows that nutrition and environment must be significant factors in addition to calving.

Continual Trauma

Repeated insults are important. Sole haemorrhage seems to disappear fairly quickly from first-calved heifers, but the scarring and other microscopic tissue changes remaining within the foot mean that they are much slower to heal if and when further attacks of laminitis occur at the second or subsequent carvings. For example, sole haemorrhages can remain for some considerable time after calving (e.g. 2–3 months) in cows, whereas first calved heifers have often recovered by this stage (27).

Breeding

Genetics plays a part in the production of lameness, both through temperament and conformation. Nervous animals are more likely to undertake sudden flight movements, tearing the hoof wall from the sole and hence weakening the white line, and are less likely to spend sufficient time lying down. Very heavy breeds seem to be more susceptible to lameness as are those animals with straight hocks, sinking pasterns, fetlocks almost touching the ground, feet turned outwards and hooves with a shallow angle of the front wall.

As inherited conformational characteristics of both feet and legs have been shown to have a significant influence on the incidence of lameness (44), bulls should be chosen with care. Suggested hoof and claw measurements are given on page 20 and in Figure 3.3. Leg conformation is less important than claw conformation in terms of heritability, as it is thought that many of the leg characteristics are the result of bad feet, rather than the cause. For example, cows which walk throwing their feet out to the side probably do so because they have overgrown claws. Excessively straight or angled hocks may lead to lameness however: an angle of 100–150 degrees seems to be ideal (44).

FOOT-BATHS

The use of foot-baths is an excellent preventive measure for lameness and cows should be walked through once or twice each week during the winter months, although some researchers (44) suggest daily usage.

Solutions of 5% formalin, 2.5% copper sulphate and zinc sulphate have all been used in routine foot-baths. Formalin is said to be beneficial in several ways:

- It draws water from the hoof, thus hardening it.
- It disinfects the heel, thus reducing heel necrosis and preventing the destabilisation of the foot which results from a sinking heel.
- It disinfects between the claws and thus helps to prevent foul and possibly also reduces the incidence of interdigital growths (i.e. skin hyperplasia—see page 49).

The activity of formalin (and most disinfectants) is influenced by temperature, a warm bath (15°C) being most effective (44).

Foot-baths will also be much more effective if cows enter with clean hooves

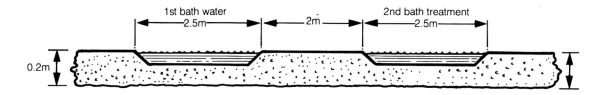

FIGURE 6.11   A dual foot-bath, the first removing dirt and debris and cleaning the feet, the second containing the active ingredient.

and are able to walk out the other side onto clean (i.e. scraped) concrete. Often two baths are used (Figure 6.11), separated by a length of raised concrete. The first bath contains water to wash off excess dirt and the raised concrete strip allows feet to drain slightly before entering the active ingredient.

Do not overfill the foot-bath – the chemical should only just cover the hoof. I have seen instances where excessively deep and concentrated formalin was used which caused burns when splashed onto the fetlock, teats and udder.

A specific antibiotic foot-bath (page 54) is used for treating digital dermatitis.

FOOT-TRIMMING

Perhaps it is appropriate to finish this book by listing foot-trimming as an important measure in the control of lameness. Although regular trimming is generally accepted as beneficial, there are surprisingly few objective studies to confirm that this is the case.

One study used a weekly system of locomotion scoring to assess the gait of cows. Cows with a score of 1 walked normally; animals with a score of 5 were acutely lame. It was found that cows which had trimmed feet walked better (viz. had a lower locomotion score) and

TABLE 6.4   The effects of hoof-trimming on lameness. Cows with trimmed feet walked better, there were fewer lame cows and fewer solar problems (44).

	Trimmed	Not Trimmed	Prob. of dliff.
Locomotion score†	1.52	1.83	**
Number of lame cows	10	15	NS
Cases of clinical lameness	23	54	***
Weeks lame for clinical cases	2.30	3.43	***
Solar problems	17	45	***

† Higher scores indicate more lameness
** $p < 0.01$; *** $p < 0.001$; NS $p > 0.05$

had a lower incidence of lameness than an equal group of cows with untrimmed feet in the same herd. The results are summarised in Table 6.4 (44). Cows with steeper claws (i.e. greater toe angle) and a shorter hoof wall walked better and developed less lameness.

In a survey of almost 2,000 feet in dairy herds in Somerset (18), 75% of the feet were found to be overgrown or misshapen, with unequal claw size being the major factor.

Cattle hoof-care is likely to be an important feature of dairy cow management in the future. Regular foot-trimming will, unfortunately, continue to feature prominently in the herdsman's daily routine.

78

References and Further Reading

Proc. BCVA = Proceedings of the British Cattle Veterinary Association
Proc. 6th Int. Symp. = Proceedings of the 6th International Symposium
Vet. Rec. = Veterinary Record
Anim. Prod. = Animal Production
J. Dairy Sci. = Journal of Dairy Science

1   ADAS (1989), *Foot Lameness in Dairy Cows*, Publication No. 3206
2   Anderson, P.H. (1990), Proc. 6th Int. Symp. on Diseases of the Ruminant Digit, Liverpool,
     p.59
3   Arkins, S. (1981), Irish Vet. Journal *35*, p.135
4   Baumgartner, C. & Distl, O. (1990), Proc. 6th Int. Symp. on Diseases of the Ruminant Digit,
     Liverpool, p.199
5   Bazeley, K. & Pinsent, P.J.N. (1984), Vet. Rec. *115*, pp.619-622
6   Bee, D.S. (1986), Proc. 5th Int. Symp. on Diseases of the Ruminant Digit, Dublin
7   Blowey, R.W. (1988), *A Veterinary Book for Dairy Farmers*, Farming Press Books, Ipswich
8   Blowey, R.W. (1990), Proc. 6th Int. Symp. on Diseases of the Ruminant Digit, Liverpool, p.55
9   Blowey, R.W. (1990), Vet. Rec. *126*, p.120
10   Blowey, R.W. (1990), Vet. Rec. *127*, pp.515-517
11   Blowey, R.W. (1992), In Practice *14*, No. 2, p.85
12   Blowey, R.W. (1992), In Practice *14*, No. 3, p.118
13   Blowey, R.W. & Sharp, M.W. (1988), Vet. Rec. *122*, p.505
14   Blowey, R.W., Sharp, M.W. & Done, S.H. (1992), Vet. Rec. *131*, p.39
15   Boosman, R. (1990), J. Vet. Medicine *37*, p.513
16   Cermak, J. (1990), Proc. 6th Int. Symp. on Diseases of the Ruminant Digit, Liverpool, p.85
17   Clarkson, D.A. & Ward, W.R. (1991), Vet. Rec. *129*, pp.511-512
18   Collick, D. (1990), Proc. 6th Int. Symp. on Diseases of the Ruminant Digit, Liverpool, p.109
19   Collick, D.W., Ward, W.R. & Dobson, H. (1989), Vet. Rec. *125*, pp.103-106
20   Colam-Ainsworth, P., Lunn, G.A., Thomas, R.C., Eddy, R.G. (1989), Vet. Rec. *125*, pp.573-575
21   David, G.P. (1990), Proc. 6th Int. Symp. on Diseases of the Ruminant Digit, Liverpool, p.1
22   Distl, O. & Mair, A. (1990), Proc. 6th Int. Symp. on Diseases of the Ruminant Digit, Liverpool,
     p.143

23   Drew, B. (1990), Bovine Medicine, p.45, edited by Andrews, Blowey, Boyd & Eddy, Blackwell Scientific Publications, Oxford
24   Eddy, R.G. & Scott, C.P. (1980), Vet. Rec. *106*, p.140
25   Esslemont, R.J. (1990), Proc. 6th Int. Symp. on Diseases of the Ruminant Digit, Liverpool, pp.237 & 276
26   Garnsworthy, P.C. & Topps, J.H. (1982), Anim. Prod. *35*, pp.113-119
27   Greenough, P.R. (1990), In Practice *12*, p.169
28   Greenough, P.R., MacCallum, F.J. & Weaver, A.D. (1981), *Lameness in Cattle*, Bristol Scientechnica
29   Hay, L. (1990), Proc. 6th Int. Symp. on Diseases of the Ruminant Digit, Liverpool, p.8
30   Hassall, S.A., Ward, W.R. & Murray, R.D. (1992), unpublished. Quoted by Ward, W.R. (1992), Proc. BCVA, July 1992, p.120
31   Hedlund, L. & Rolls, J. (1977), J. Dairy Sci. *50*, pp.1807-1812
32   Hughes, J. (1990), *The Cow and her Cubicle*, Proc. 6th Int. Symp. on Diseases of the Ruminant Digit, Liverpool, p.276
33   Hughes, J. (1992), Proc. BCVA, Wye, Kent, p.43
34   Kameya, Y., Yamada, H., Abe, N. & Matsuda, A. (1990), supplementary paper to Proc. 6th Int. Symp. on Diseases of the Ruminant Digit, Liverpool, published in Proc. BCVA 1990-91, p.7
35   Kelly, J.M. (1990), *Data from University of Edinburgh/Dalgety Spillers Dairy Herd Health & Productivity Scheme 1987-90*
36   Kempson, S. & Logue, D.N. (1993), Vet. Rec., (in press)
37   Leonard, N., O'Connell, J. & O'Farrell, K. (1992), Proc. 7th Int. Symp. on Diseases of the Ruminant Digit, Denmark
38   Livesey, C.T. (1984), Vet. Rec. *114*, p.22
39   Livesey, C.T. & Flemming, F.L. (1984), Vet. Rec. *114*, p.510
40   Logue, D.N., Bradley, H. & Kempson, S. (1990), supplementary paper to Proc. 6th Int. Symp. on Diseases of the Ruminant Digit, Liverpool, published in Proc. BCVA 1990-91, p.38
41   Maclean, C.W. (1965), Vet. Rec. *77*, p.662
42   Manson, F.D. & Leaver, J.D. (1988), Anim. Prod. *47*, pp.191-199
43   Manson, F.D. & Leaver, J.D. (1989), Anim. Prod. *49*, pp.15-22
44   McDaniel, B.T. & Wilk, J.C. (1990), supplementary paper to Proc. 6th Int. Symp. on Diseases of the Ruminant Digit, Liverpool, published in Proc. BCVA 1990-91, p.66
45   Mortellaro, C. (1990), personal communication
46   Nilsson, S.A. (1963), Acten. Vet. Scand., Vol. 4, supplement No. 1
47   O'Connell, J.M., Meany, M.J. & Giller, P.S. (1991), Irish Vet. J. *44*, pp.8-13
48   Peterse, D.J. (1992), *Foot Lameness*, Bovine Medicine, p.353, edited by Andrews, Blowey, Boyd & Eddy, Blackwell Scientific Publications, Oxford
49   Peterse, D.J., Korver, S., Oldenbroek, J.K., Talmon, F.P. (1984), Vet. Rec. *115*, p.629
50   Potter, M.J. & Broom, D.M. (1990), Proc. 6th Int. Symp. on Diseases of the Ruminant Digit, Liverpool, p.80
51   Ral, R. (1990), Proc. 6th Int. Symp. on Diseases of the Ruminant Digit, Liverpool, p.219
52   Read, D.H., Walker, R.E., Castro, A.E., Sundberg, J.P., Thermond, M.C. (1992), Vet. Rec. *130*, p.60
53   Rowlands, G.J., Russell, A.M., Williams, L.A. (1983), Vet. Rec. *113*, p.441
54   Rowlands, G.J., Russell, A.M., Williams, L.A. (1985), Vet. Rec. *117*, pp.576-580
55   Russell, A.M., Rowlands, G.J., Shaw, S.R. & Weaver, A.D. (1982), Vet. Rec. *111*, pp.155-165
56   Singh, S.S., Ward, W.R. & Murray, R.D. (1993), Vet. Bulletin (in press)
57   Sumner, J. (1989), *Design and Maintenance of Housing Systems*, Proc. Brit. Mastitis Conference, Stoneleigh, p.10
58   Toussaint Raven, E. (1985), *Cattle Footcare and Claw Trimming*, Farming Press Books, Ipswich
59   Vermont, J.J. & Leach, D.H. (1990), supplementary paper to Proc. 6th Int. Symp. on Diseases of the Ruminant Digit, Liverpool, published in Proc. BCVA 1990-91, p.4
60   Ward, W.R. (1992), Proc. BCVA, Wye, Kent, p.120
61   Whitaker, D.M., Kelly, J.M. & Smith, E.J. (1983), Vet. Rec. *113*, pp.60-62
62   Wierenga, H.K. & Hopster, H. (1990), Appl. Anim. Behav. Sci. 26, p.309

63   Giltspur UK Ltd (Cowslips), 13 Calhame Road, Ballyclare, Co. Antrim BT39 9NA, UK
64   Demotec, Brentanostrasse 21, D6369, Nidderau 1, Germany

FURTHER READING

Blowey, R.W. (1988) *A Veterinary Book for Dairy Farmers*, Farming Press, Ipswich

Blowey, R.W. & Edmondson, P. (1995), *Mastitis Control in Dairy Herds*, chapter 8, Farming Press, Ipswich

Blowey, R.W. & Weaver, A.D. (1991), *A Colour Atlas of Diseases and Disorders of Cattle,* Wolfe Publications, London

Greenough, P.R., MacCullum, F.J. & Weaver, A.D. (1981), *Lameness in Cattle*, Bristol Scientechnica

Greenough, P.R. & Weaver, A.D. (1977), *Lameness in Cattle*, W.B. Saunders & Co.

Ossent, P. (1995), 'The Pathology of Digital Disease' in *Cattle Practice*, vol. 3, p. 263.

Phillips, C.J.C. (1993), *Cattle Behaviour*, Farming Press Books, Ipswich

Tranter, W.P. (1992), *The Epidemiology and Control of Lameness in Pasture-fed Dairy Cattle*, a thesis presented to Massey University, New Zealand

Weaver, A.D. (1986), *Bovine Surgery and Lameness*, Blackwell Scientific Publications, Oxford

Index

Page numbers in italics refer to figures or plates.

FARMING PRESS BOOKS & VIDEOS

Below is a sample from the wide range of agricultural and veterinary books and videos we publish. For more information or for a free illustrated catalogue of all our publications please contact:

Farming Press
Miller Freeman plc
Wharfedale Road, Ipswich IP1 4LG, United Kingdom
Telephone (01473) 241122   Fax (01473) 240501

Also by Roger Blowey

A Veterinary Book for Dairy Farmers has achieved worldwide recognition as an authoritative and usable guide.

It deals with the full range of cattle ailments grouped broadly according to the age and development of the animal from the young calf to the adult cow. The emphasis of the book is on the causes and prevention of cattle diseases, particularly where husbandry measures can be applied as a means of control. Detailed, lucid, full of illustrations, *A Veterinary Book for Dairy Farmers* is an essential tool in the daily fight to keep intensively managed livestock in first-class condition.

Associated with *Cattle Lameness and Hoofcare* is a 55 minute video *Footcare in Cattle: Hoof Structure & Trimming*, written and presented by Roger Blowey. The first half of the video contains a clear demonstration of hoof anatomy using specially prepared laboratory specimens. Roger Blowey shows the process of hoof overgrowth and how this contributes to cow discomfort and ailments such as sole ulcers.

After relating the theory of trimming to hoof anatomy, Roger Blowey then goes on to the farm to demonstrate basic foot trimming.

Cattle Ailments   EDDIE STRAITON
The recognition and treatment of all the common cattle ailments shown in over 300 photographs.

Cattle Behaviour   CLIVE PHILLIPS
Describes what cattle do and why – what is normal in young and old, male and female, and what is not.

Cattle Feeding   JOHN OWEN
A detailed account of the principles and practices of cattle feeding, including optimal diet formulation.

Cattle Footcare and Claw Trimming
E TOUSSAINT RAVEN
Combines a guide to the causes, progress, treatment and prevention of foot ailments with practical details on claw trimming.

Calf Rearing
THICKETT, MITCHELL, HALLOWS
Covers the housed rearing of calves to twelve weeks, reflecting modern experience in a wide variety of situations.

Calving the Cow and Care of the Calf
EDDIE STRAITON
A highly illustrated manual offering practical, commonsense guidance.

The Herdsman's Book
MALCOLM STANSFIELD
The stockperson's guide to the dairy enterprise.

Mastitis Control in Dairy Herds
ROGER BLOWEY, PETER EDMONDSON
An in-depth account of all aspects of mastitis from physiology to the impact of machine milking on prevention and treatment.

Farming Press is a division of Miller Freeman plc, which provides a wide range of media services in agriculture and allied businesses. Among the magazines published by the group are *Arable Farming*, *Dairy Farmer*, *Farming News*, and *Pig Farming*. For a specimen copy contact the address above.